COMPLEX REGIONAL PAIN SYNDROME (CRPS):

PATIENTS' PERSPECTIVE OF LIVING IN CHRONIC PAIN
Volume V

Alaa Abd-Elsayed M.D., MPH, FASA and Eric M. Phillips

D1534075

First edition, 2021 – Volume V

ISBN:

Other books published by authors:

Alaa Abd-Elsayed

- Chronic Pain: The Patient and Family Journey
- If the Savior is not Safe, How Can He Save?
- Pain: A Review Guide
- Infusion Therapy for Pain, Headache and Related Conditions
- Complex Regional Pain Syndrome (CRPS): Patients' Perspective of Living in Chronic Pain: Volume 1
- Complex Regional Pain Syndrome (CRPS): Patients' Perspective of Living in Chronic Pain: Volume 1-Picture eBook
- Complex Regional Pain Syndrome (CRPS): Patients' Perspective of Living in Chronic Pain: Volume II
- Complex Regional Pain Syndrome (CRPS): Patients' Picture eBook Guide: Volume II
- What is CRPS? A Helpful Guide to Teach Children About Complex Regional Pain Syndrome (CRPS): Volume III
- Complex Regional Pain Syndrome (CRPS) and Amputation: A Patients' Picture eBook Guide: Volume III
- Complex Regional Pain Syndrome (CRPS) and Amputation: A Difficult Decision to Make: Volume IV.

Eric M. Phillips

- Complex Regional Pain Syndrome (CRPS): Patients' Perspective of Living in Chronic Pain: Volume 1
- Complex Regional Pain Syndrome (CRPS): Patients' Perspective of Living in Chronic Pain: Volume 1-Picture eBook
- Don't Diet: Change Your Eating Habits - Proper Eating for Good Health
- Complex Regional Pain Syndrome (CRPS): Patients' Perspective of Living in Chronic Pain: Volume II
- Complex Regional Pain Syndrome (CRPS): Patients' Picture eBook Guide: Volume II
- What is CRPS? A Helpful Guide to Teach Children About Complex Regional Pain Syndrome (CRPS): Volume III
- Complex Regional Pain Syndrome (CRPS) and Amputation: A Patients' Picture eBook Guide: Volume III
- Complex Regional Pain Syndrome (CRPS) and Amputation: A Difficult Decision to Make: Volume IV.

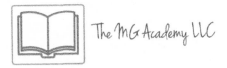 The MG Academy LLC

Dedication

To my parents, my wife and my two beautiful kids Maro and George.

To all CRPS patients.

Alaa Abd-Elsayed

Dedication

To my loving parents, Janet and my late father Leonard (Lenny) for all their love, and support.

To my beautiful and supportive wife Mercedes, her three children and her grandson.

To my mentor, teacher and greatest friend the late Doctor Hooshang Hooshmand.

To all CRPS patients worldwide.

Eric M. Phillips

TABLE OF CONTENTS

Preface

First, I would like to thank all patients who shared their personal stories with CRPS in this book. We recently published the first volume, which included the stories of several patients who live suffering from CRPS. When we talk about suffering, it is not only pain, but suffering made some patients commit suicide or have an amputation to get rid of the pain.

CRPS is a very serious condition and dealing with it otherwise is not wise. Unfortunately, there is a huge lack of knowledge even among health care providers about the seriousness of this condition and what it can lead to if not managed quickly and aggressively. Early and aggressive management can lead to control and even cure of the pain, but lack of diagnosis and not understanding the urgency of treating this condition can lead to a worsening of pain with associated depression, anxiety, limb atrophy, amputation, and potential suicide.

My friend Eric, and I authored volumes I, II III, and IV of this book series, to share the stories of patients suffering from CRPS. Our goal is to increase public awareness of the severity of this condition. What we mean by the public is everyone from employers, spouses, health care providers, and others. It is very important to provide support to CRPS patients to avoid the serious consequences of the condition. Employers should understand the limitations of their employees; "yes, the condition can cause pain to touch," spouses need to support their partners with CRPS, and health care providers should treat it aggressively and quickly. If they have limited experience treating this condition, then they should immediately refer the patient to the experts.

With CRPS, we are racing against time, and providers should start with a non-pharmacological treatment, then medications, and if they fail, then interventions. If one modality is not working, health care providers should move to the next modality without waiting. They should discuss a plan with the patient, with one step after another, and this depends on the success or failure of different modalities.

I hope this book will help increase public awareness about the condition and help CRPS patients to understand the seriousness of this condition and the need to seek help as soon as possible without waiting for too long.

Alaa Abd-Elsayed, MD, MPH, FASA

Preface

I would like to especially thank all the CRPS patients for taking the time to write and share their personal stories. It is generous of all of you to share your journey of living with this painful disease in this book. Your willingness to share your story will provide great help and support to others who are suffering from CRPS.

I have been working in the CRPS community for over 32-years to help advocate for other CRPS patients. As, being a sufferer of CRPS for over the past 35-years, and being an amputee for 13-years, I understand the struggles and pain that CRPS patients endure. The biggest downfall for most patients is the lack of understanding of CRPS by the medical community, and the public.

I have been fortunate to know and work with my friend Doctor Alaa Abd-Elsayed over the years. It has been a great honor for me to work on this fifth book with Doctor Al, and all the patients that were so gracious enough to submit their stories.

We both felt that writing this book that shared patient's personal stories of living life as an Amputee with CRPS would help to continue spreading the desperately needed awareness, help educate the public and the medical community that CRPS is a real and serious disease.

I hope this book will be helpful and provide reassurance to other CRPS patients that they are not alone; with their daily battle of dealing with the chronic pain of CRPS. Moreover, I also hope this book will help the medical community worldwide to understand how patients live and cope with this unrelenting painful disease. Remember, we all have to work together to help spread awareness in finding a cure for CRPS.

Eric M. Phillips

INTRODUCTION

Alaa Abd-Elsayed, MD, MPH, FASA, and Eric M. Phillips

Complex regional pain syndrome (CRPS), is a poorly understood condition by the medical community. Many patients may suffer long before getting diagnosed or even receive proper treatment.

CRPS is a painful disease that affects the patient physically, mentally, and emotionally. To obtain a complete understanding of this disease, one must read the patient's personal story to get a sense of what can potentially happen to some patients.

As we are all well aware of CRPS is a complex disease to diagnose, treat, and to understand. Treating physicians must take into consideration that each patient is affected differently by CRPS due to the different stages of the disease. The patient and treating physician need to work as a team to create a proper treatment plan that will help the patient control their pain.

CRPS has become a global disease, with millions of cases worldwide. CRPS affects patients in the same way. It does not matter if the patient lives in the United States, Australia, Britain, France or anywhere else in the world. Every CRPS patient suffers from the same chronic pain and has difficulty in receiving proper treatment. Unfortunately, CRPS patients must fight daily to deal with their pain and try to get the recognition that CRPS is an actual disease.

We have created this book to help share how patients suffer from the pain of CRPS. Until a doctor, relative, or friend sees the damage that CRPS causes, one cannot comprehend the pain patients deal with daily. These stories you will read in this book range from patients having early stages of the disease to the end-stage of the disease.

Our main goal for this book is to help spread awareness about CRPS. Educating the medical community on the topic of CRPS is a high priority. The medical community needs to understand how devastating CRPS is and how it affects the patient physically, mentally, and emotionally.

*In this volume we are including a new section in the book. In this new section, we will share updated stories from patients who have previously submitted their story, in past volumes of this book series to update us on how they are doing since their original story was published.

CAN COMPLEX REGIONAL PAIN SYNDROME (CRPS) SPREAD?
THE ANSWER IS YES

Eric M. Phillips
International RSD Foundation
www.rsdinfo.com

Abstract. Complex regional pain syndrome (CRPS) is a complex and disabling disease caused by a minor injury or trauma. Patients suffer for years with either constant burning pain or an ice-cold pain in their effected extremity. In some cases of CRPS, the patient will experience spread of the disease from one limb to another, whole body spread, spread to the face, or develop internal organ involvement. There have been reports of other complications associated with the spread of the disease, such as visual disturbance and cardiac disturbance, etc......

A majority of physicians do not understand or believe that CRPS can spread. There is a great need for more research into the development of spread in CRPS patients.

Keywords: Complex regional pain syndrome (CRPS), internal organ spread, and spread of CRPS.

Introduction

For decades there has been a misconception among the medical community if CRPS can spread? The answer to this important question is undoubtedly yes, it can spread in a majority of CRPS patients.

There have been many published reports by some of the great pioneers in the field of CRPS.

The phenomenon of spread in CRPS patients have been reported by Doctors Hooshmand, Schwartzman, Veldman, Maleki, Kozin, and Radt, and many others (1-6).

In this chapter, I will discuss how CRPS can spread. Spread of CRPS can be caused by many factors, such as surgery (amputation, carpal tunnel, tarsal tunnel, and thoracic outlet syndrome), cryotherapy (the application of ice), improper treatment, and failed procedures. These are just a few examples of how CRPS can spread.

Spread of CRPS

In the research work done by my mentor the late Doctor Hooshmand, he believed that CRPS is not usually limited to one part of an extremity or in one extremity.

Usually, the pathological sympathetic function spreads to adjacent areas of the body (1,7).

In CRPS the sympathetic nerves follow the path of the blood vessels rather than somatic nerve roots resulting in thermotomal rather than dermatomal sensory nerve distribution (mistaken for hysterical sensory loss) may cause a complex clinical picture that baffles the clinician and forces the clinician to blame the patient as being hysterical, hypochondriac, and blaming the serious warning signs of CRPS as "functional and not "organic". Then the patient is sent to the psychiatrist who tries to shut the patient up with strong tranquilizers, benzodiazepams, with further disastrous results by aggravating the patients CRPS due to inactivity (7).

The sympathetic nervous system is complex, bilateral, and diffuse. Its job is alerting the mechanism to alert the entire body against stress and its manifestations are complex and multifaceted (7).

The usual factors facilitating the spread of the disease are surgical procedures, application of ice, and stress of too much activity or inactivity (8). In Doctor Hooshmand's study of 824 CRPS patients, the number one aggravator was cryosurgery, followed by surface cryotherapy (application of ice) applied for more than two months. The surface cryotherapy less than two months did not show the tendency for spread of CRPS (7-10).

Cryosurgery, similar to radiofrequency surgery, does not limit the freezing damage to a circumscribed nerve. The concentric field of freezing cannot limit itself to a small anatomical target. Damage to the adjacent normal nerves contribute to spread and expansion of the lesion (7,9).

Spread of CRPS can develop in any of the first three stages of the disease (1,3,5,6,10,11).

The research by Kozin et al., shows that CRPS can spread vertically or horizontally in both upper or both lower extremities (5,10). Also, undergoing any surgical procedure can promote the potential spread of CRPS (6,7,10). Maleki, et al., published a retrospective analysis of 27 CRPS patients. In this study, all 27 patients had experienced a spread of their pain (4,10).

8

In Doctor Hooshmand's textbook on CRPS, he reported the chain of sympathetic ganglia from the base of the skull to sacral regions on the right and left sides, typically spread the pathologic impulse to other extremities (1,7).

The observed phenomenon of referred pain of CRPS can sometimes be mistaken for the spread of the disease. These are two separate issues that patients go through (7,10).

The spread of CRPS is not usually limited to one part of an extremity or one extremity. Usually, the pathological sympathetic function spreads to adjacent areas (1,11). CRPS can also spread to the oral facial region; it causes necrosis (death of cells) of the maxillary and mandibular bones in the areas of the root canals (11).

In the late stages of CRPS, due to prolonged immobilization, or improper treatment such as unnecessary surgery or application of ice, the disease shows a tendency to spread (11). The spread of CRPS may be vertical from arm to leg (or vice versa) on the same side or may be horizontal from arm to arm or leg to leg. The spread which occurs in about one third of patients is more likely to develop after surgical procedure (1,2,8,9,11-18).

The mechanism of spread is due to the fact that at the level of the spinal cord, the sympathetic input has a tendency to cross the midline to the opposite side. The second reason for spread is a chain of relay stations of the sympathetic nerves in the form of sympathetic ganglia on each side of the spine (11,17).

The main reason for the CRPS becoming bilateral and spreading to other extremities is because in contrast to the somatic nervous system, the sympathetic nervous system has bilateral innervation. In the somatic nervous system (usual sensation and motor function) the abnormalities in dermatome in a specific nerve root distribution, whereas in CRPS the abnormality is distributed among the blood vessels, distribution of nerves (Thermatomes) and to the sympathetic ganglia and then across the midline collections, the condition reflects itself on both sides rather than one side of the body. This bilateral manifestation through the sympathetic plexi across the midline explains the patient's problem with headache, dizziness, tinnitus, chest pain, and abdominal manifestations of CRPS (gastritis, diarrhea, cramps) and spread of CRPS to other extremities (11).

Surgery as a Cause of Spread in CRPS

As, I wrote in our second CRPS book, many physicians have the misconception that surgery is safe for CRPS patients. This is another false and misleading misconception that will cause the patient more harm. Surgery can cause more harm and spread of the disease. Patients need to avoid any unnecessary surgery due to the high risk that their CRPS will spread and cause more pain (10).

Over the years working with Doctor Hooshmand, we have seen the spread of the disease in patients who have undergone surgical sympathectomy (be it surgical, chemical, or radiofrequency). Any type of sympathectomy is useless for advanced cases of CRPS. It will cause a rapid spread of CRPS to other parts of the body and cause more pain for the patient (10).

Surgery for the infusion pump or the spinal cord stimulator (SCS) also causes the spread of the disease. These implants are apt to fail and cause more pain, and spread of the disease for the patient (10).

In Doctor Hooshmand's review article of 824 CRPS cases, he states there are times that surgery is unavoidable (8). Examples: tear of a ligament or cartilage in the knee joint that would preclude weight-bearing. In such patients, epidural nerve block with a combination of Bupivacaine and 20 to 30 mg Prednisolone before, during, and after surgery (with the help of an epidural catheter) helps reduce the side effects of surgical trauma. Another example is an extensor deformity of a finger, causing a useless hand, which in turn aggravates CRPS (8,10). Elective surgery for presumptive conditions such as carpal tunnel, tarsal tunnel, and thoracic outlet syndrome(TOS)- in spite of normal nerve conduction studies - only adds a new source of neuropathic pain at the surgical scar. According to Cherington, et al, there is a tendency for unnecessary TOS surgery, elective surgery is the strongest predictor (P<0.001) of poor treatment outcome (7,19).

According to Rowbotham, "amputation is not to be recommended as pain therapy (7,20)."

Doctor Hooshmand reported that 11 patients in his series of 824 CRPS patients who underwent amputation showed marked deterioration post-op (7,8). The surgical stump was the source of multiple neuromas with sever CRPS II type of intractable pain. Amputation should be avoided by all means due to its side effects of aggravation of pain and tendency for spread of CRPS (7,8).

The commonest forms of surgical procedures that cause permanent damage and permanent intractability of CRPS are (21):

- Carpal tunnel surgery.

- Tarsal tunnel surgery.
- Rotator cuff surgery.
- Ulnar nerve decompression.
- Surgical exploration of the knee, neuroma, or ankle.
- Thoracic outlet syndrome surgery.
- Removal of a bulging disc or herniated discs in the distribution of spasm and pain secondary to CRPS.

Patients and physicians must have an open line of communication when the topic of having unnecessary surgery is discussed. Having any type of surgery can be a high risk for any CRPS patient. It is better to have all the facts in place before having any surgery that could potentially spread the CRPS. Avoiding surgery can help spare the patient from the unwanted spread of the disease (10).

Internal Organ Complications in CRPS

Another complication of CRPS is spread of the disease into internal organs. Doctors Hooshmand, Schwartzman, and Veldman are just few of a handful of doctors who have reported cases of CRPS affecting the internal organs in CRPS patients (7,11,18,22).

CRPS invariably involves the internal organs. Usually, the skin surface is cold at the expense of increased circulation to the internal organs. This increased circulation can cause osteoporosis, fractures of bone, abdominal cramps and diarrhea, disturbance of absorption of foods with resultant weight loss, water retention with aggravation of premenstrual headaches and depression, persistent nausea and vomiting, as well as severe vascular headaches mistaken for "cluster headache" (11). In addition, CRPS can

12

cause the complication of intractable hypertension which responds best to alpha I blockers (Dibenzyline, Hytrin, or Clonodine). CRPS can cause attacks of irregular or fast heart-beat, chest pain, coronary artery spasm (angina), as well as disturbance of function of other internal organs (11).

A few other examples are frequency and urgency of urination, respiratory disturbance such as dyspnea and apneic attacks, and attacks of severe abdominal pain (11).

Attacks of swelling of the internal organs complicated by intermittent constriction of the blood vessels to different organs can result in chest pain, attacks of sharp central pain (stabbing severe pain in the chest or abdomen), and changes in the patient's voice (suddenly developing a temporary "chipmunk" type of voice change). The sharp, stabbing, central pain can be helped with treatment with medications such as anticonvulsant (Tegretol or Neurontin) (11).

The internal organs complication may become aggravated by the traumatic effect of sympathetic nerve blocks. One such complication is accidental trauma to the kidney with resultant hematuria (blood in urine) and aggravation of hypertension (11).

Because of the above complex phenomenon, in CRPS the sympathetic nerves follow the path of the blood vessels rather than somatic nerve roots resulting thermotomal rather than dermatomal sensory nerve distribution (mistaken for hysterical sensory loss) may cause a complex clinical picture that baffles the clinician and forces the clinician to blame the patient as being hysterical, hypochondriac, and blaming the serious warning signs of CRPS complications as "functional and not organic"(11).

13

The end result is the deadly phrase **"it is all in your head"** which practically almost all CRPS patients have heard and had to deal with in the course of their treatment. The patient's symptoms and signs are real and they are not a figment of their imagination. The treating physician needs to take the time to learn and understand that the sympathetic system is complex, bilateral and diffuse (11).

Other Complications Caused by CRPS

Over the last few decades many CRPS patients have developed many other complications that are associated with CRPS.

These complications should not be ignored by the treating physician. These complications should be address and treated in a timely fashion. The CRPS patient suffers enough from the daily pain of the disease. They do not need to suffer from other complications.

As Doctor Hooshmand and I have reported in the article titled Various Complications of CRPS, we found most patients suffer from the standard signs and symptoms of CRPS (10,11). Over time a majority of patients that have suffered for many years to decades do develop various complications of the disease. Over the years we have recognized a large array of various complications associated with CRPS which often go untreated. Many of these complications are not well recognized by the medical community. However, CRPS continues to be a very complex disease to understand and to treat. These various complications can impede the proper treatment for the spread of the disease and the underlying issues that arise from these complications (10,11).

It is well known that during the long duration of the disease when patients reach stage IV, they start to develop various complications such as disturbance of the immune system (neurogenic inflammation), limbic system, cardiac system, the endocrine system, and the respiratory system. These are just a few of the various complications of CRPS (11).

Below is a list of other complications that are associated with CRPS. Few physicians recognized these complications (1,8,11,22,23).

List of Complications in CRPS:

- Agitation
- Cardiac Disturbance
- Depression
- Disturbance of the Immune System
- Disturbance of Judgment
- Dysphagia
- Endocrine System Dysfunction
- Fatigue
- Gardner Diamond Syndrome (Spontaneous Bruising)
- Gastrointestinal Complications
- GERDS
- Headaches (Migraine)
- Hearing Complications
- Hypothyroidism
- Insomnia
- Internal Organ Involvement
- Interstitial Cystitis
- Intractable Hypertension
- Keratitis Sicca (Dry Eyes)

- Limbic System Dysfunction
- Low Cortisol Levels
- Movement Disorders
- Respiratory System Complications
- Skin Lesions, Rashes, and Ulcers
- Spread of CRPS
- Tinnitus
- Urological Complications
- Visual Disturbance
- Vulvodynia

Cardiac Complications in CRPS

In my time working with Doctor Hooshmand at his clinic, we had seen many CRPS patients who had developed cardiac complications. Chest pain due to CRPS is quite common due to the fact that the cardiac sympathetic plexus surrounding the heart is a rich sympathetic nerve structure, and its dysfunction can cause severe chest pain. CRPS causes three independent negative influences on cardiac function (11).

1.The sympathetic system is responsible for three main functions, i.e., temperature regulation, vital signs, and regulation of the immune system. The vital signs in the form of heart beat, blood pressure and respiration are up regulated and accelerated by stimulation of the sympathetic system. The CRPS is not a simple hyperactivity only stimulation of the sympathetic system. It is the result of dysfunction of the sympathetic system. This dysfunction shows instability of the sympathetic system at times causing fluctuation of blood pressure and at other times causing attacks of fast heart-beat (11).

2. The second reason CRPS affects cardiac function is due to the anatomical innervation of the heart muscles. Of all the visceral organs, the heart has the richest innervation of the sympathetic system. This is in the form of cardiac plexus which is a rich plexus of nerves surrounding the heart. In any stressful condition, the natural response is rapid heart-beat and rise of the blood pressure. The CRPS being a distressful type of dysfunction of the sympathetic system, results in repetitive pathological and exaggerated response of the sympathetic system to stress, chest pain, palpation, and bouts of high blood pressure (11).

3. One of the main principles of development of CRPS is inflammation. CRPS is a condition with four major features. First, the allodynia and hyperpathia is typical with pains seen with sympathetic dysfunction. Second, is motor response to such pain in the form of vasoconstriction, muscle spasm and muscle tremor. Thirdly, inflammation in the form of skin rash, swelling of soft tissues in the extremities, increased circulation in the visceral structures resulting in osteoporosis, pelvic inflammation, and attacks of vascular headaches. The same inflammation and increased visceral circulation cause distress on the heart (11).

Obviously if the patient has already had pre-existing cardiac disease, the distressful disease of CRPS is going to cause further stress on the heart on the basis of the above mentioned three principles (11).

Another symptom that we have seen associated with the cardiac complications of CRPS is a rash across the patient's chest wall (11).

Rasmussen and colleagues have reported that atypical chest pain is a common complaint in 94 % of CRPS patients (11,24,25).

17

Smith and colleagues published an article reporting that pre-syncope and syncope are complications in lower limb CRPS patients. These symptoms are related to autonomic dysfunction. In their study they reported 40% of CRPS patients showed symptoms of pre-syncope and syncope (11,26).

Unfortunately, cardiac complications of CRPS go unnoticed and untreated, which does not help the patient. These patients are blamed as being neurotic especially due to the fact that many CRPS patients are young and they have no coronary artery disease.

Limbic System Complications in CRPS

CRPS can also cause complications with the limbic system. According to Benarroch, the neuropathic pain of CRPS is regional, and its polysynaptic sensory fibers terminate bilaterally in the limbic system (11,27).

This explains the symptoms of insomnia, agitation, irritability and depression in CRPS (8,11,28). Practically every patient suffering from CRPS demonstrates some degree of limbic system disturbance. These patients are expected to be depressed in more than 3/4 of the cases, anxious in practically every one of the cases, and to suffer from insomnia, agitation, irritability and poor judgment in practically every one of the cases. These manifestations are one of the four criteria for the diagnosis of CRPS. There is no way the limbic system can be left intact in the face of CRPS (11).

Skin Lesions and Skin Rash Complications in CRPS

Another frequent complication seen in some CRPS patients are skin lesions and skin rashes.

A few years after onset of CRPS, the patient can develop neurodermatitis, trophic ulcers, Gardner-Diamond Syndrome (GDS) (spontaneous bruising), and skin rashes (11,24,29,30). Doctor Goris has reported that 5% of patients with long-standing CRPS develop various skin problems that are very difficult to heal (11,31). Trophic ulcers are not unusual in CRPS, being a sympathetic nervous system dysfunction, it manifests itself as follows:

- Hyperpathic and allodynic pain (pain accompanied by change in vital signs, sweating and pain that becomes worse with simple touch or a breeze) (11).

- The response to the pain is in the form of motor response the spinal cord resulting in constriction of blood vessels, cold extremities, and muscle spasm, tremor and flexion deformity (11).

This disturbance of the immune system manifests in inflammation, spontaneous bruising and black and blue spots over the skin, neurodermatitis, edema and swelling that mimic- conditions such as carpal tunnel and tarsal tunnel syndrome. In addition, the immune system disturbance in more severe cases not only cause neurodermatitis, but also causes trophic ulcers. Trophic ulcers usually develop after treatment with cast immobilization, wheelchair immobilization, surgical treatment or application of ice. At, times, the trophic ulcer and immune system disturbance are caused by incomplete pain management (11).

It's important that these skin lesions and rashes should be address and treated as soon as possible to help prevent further spread and added pain for the patient.

19

Urological Complications in CRPS

Another complication that is seen in many CRPS patients is urological complications.

In severe and chronic stages of sympathetic dysfunction, neuroinflammation results in interstitial cystitis, pelvic inflammatory disease (PID) and sterile abscess (11,32).

Chancellor, and colleagues have reported urological complication in 25% of CRPS patients (11,22,33). The International Association for the Study of Pain calls interstitial cystitis as a form of CRPS (11,34).

According to Galloway et al., interstitial cystitis might be a form of CRPS, in which the target organ is the urinary bladder. They also reported a similarity between the clinical course of CRPS and interstitial cystitis (11,32).

Gastrointestinal Complications in CRPS

Many patients also develop gastrointestinal (GI) complications such as GERD 73% and Dysphagia in 17% as reported by Schwartzman (11,24).

Other complications are diarrhea, irritable bowel syndrome (IBS), and severe constipation seen in 90% of CRPS patients (7,11,24). Intestine and Bowel complications are often the signs of inflammation in CRPS. This is very similar to the same inflammation that involves the extremities.

Hearing and Visual Complications in CRPS

There are some patients who have experienced issues with their hearing and vision. These are other complication that are associated with CRPS.

Hyperacusis is a condition associated with painful sensations to sound. De Klaver et al. reported that 38% of patients with CRPS related dystonia had symptoms of hyperacusis. Doctor De Klaver and his group found that hyperacusis is common among patients suffering with CRPS related dystonia. Hyperacusis in these patients may reflect the spreading of central sensitization, to auditory circuitry (11,35).

CRPS patients frequently develop blurring of vision, reading difficulty, problem with focusing, and dizziness in the form of vertiginous attacks (either the body or the objects moving around). As well as hearing problems such as buzzing in the ear (tinnitus) (11).

It is immaterial which part of the body has had the damage causing CRPS. As the sympathetic nervous system is intermingled and connected through sympathetic ganglia which are on each side of the vertebrae from lower cervical spine region all the way down to the tailbone. This chain of sympathetic connections causes the spread of CRPS to symptoms and signs both across the midline of the opposite side (from hand to hand or from foot to foot) and vertically up and down the spine. As a result, the patient may have CRPS due to a knee injury or injury to the foot or hand and yet may develop stimulation and abnormal function of the sympathetic system causing constriction of the blood vessels to the brain. When the blood vessels are constricted in the distribution of vertebral arteries in the cervical spine and in the distribution of the blood vessels providing circulation for the hearing center and brainstem, the patient develops attacks of dizziness, trouble with focusing with the eyes (due to brainstem dysfunction which has the responsibility of coordinating the eye movements), and buzzing in the ears (tinnitus) (11).

21

At times the original injury that has caused CRPS may cause retinal detachment (damage to the retina of the eye) or bleeding of the eye. For this reason, the patient should have a careful eye examination by an ophthalmologist as well. Proper cervical, paravertebral and epidural blocks can help correct the above symptoms. Keratitis Sicca which is due to CRPS at early stage causing pain and irritation in the eye with secondary excessive secretion tears. As the condition becomes chronic, the tear glands become exhausted, causing "dry eye" (Keratitis Sicca) (11).

Conclusion

The phenomenon of spread in CRPS has been debated and reported for decades. CRPS is a complex disease to diagnose and treat. Over time a majority of patients develop spread of the disease, and also develop other complications that most physicians do not recognize or understand how to treat it.

Over the years there have been many published reports that back up this theory that CRPS can spread, and cause other various complications to patients suffering from this painful disease (1,8,10-18).

Spread of the disease, and the other complications of CRPS should be taken seriously by the medical community. CRPS patients suffer enough with their pain. Their suffering becomes worse when the disease spreads to another limb, internally, and when they develop other complications from the disease.

In some CRPS cases the development of spread is cause by surgery and improper treatment. There are cases where the patients develop spread on its own due to the duration of the disease and from the lack of treatment.

Physicians must remember that there are patients who suffer from CRPS for many years, and they may not develop spread of the disease. These patients are fortunate that their symptoms stay in one limb. This should not discount the fact that the disease can spread for a majority of patients.

Physicians who treat CRPS patients should not overlook or dismiss the fact CRPS can spread to other parts of the body or into the internal organs (7,10). Avoiding any unnecessary surgeries, and the application of ice helps prevent the spread of CRPS. (8-10). If the symptoms of spread are present, the physician should provide the proper treatment with nerve blocks, strong non-addicting pain medications, antidepressants, and nonsteroidal anti-inflammatory medications to help treat the new symptoms caused by the spread of the disease (10).

In regards to treatment, Doctor Hooshmand believed when treating CRPS patients, if their opposite extremity looks normal, the treatment should be given to both extremities because of the principle of bilateral innervation.

More research, education, and awareness are needed on the subject of spread of CRPS. Countless patients suffer daily. When the disease spreads it creates more pain for the patient, and the lack of proper treatment by the treating physician to help control the spread of the disease will cause the patient more unwanted pain and suffering.

Dedication

I would like to dedicate this chapter to my mentor the late Doctor Hooshang Hooshmand and the late Doctor Robert J. Schwartzman. We owe both Doctors a debt of gratitude for all their dedication to help and treat CRPS patients, and for their amazing research work in the field of CRPS.

They were both great Neurologist and great teachers. We have lost two great pioneers that dedicated their life to help and educate the CRPS community.

We should acknowledge that they both helped bring a greater awareness to a disease that is so difficult to diagnose and treat.

Both Doctors provided the answer to the question can CRPS spread? The answer is Yes!

I personally thank both doctors for all their dedication to help others in pain.

References

1. Hooshmand H. Chronic Pain: Reflex Sympathetic Dystrophy: Prevention and Management. CRC Press, Boca Raton FL. 1993.

2. Schwartzman RJ. Reflex sympathetic dystrophy. Handbook of Clinical Neurology. Spinal Cord Trauma, H.L. Frankel, editor. Elsevier Science Publisher B.V. 1992; 17: 121-136.

3. Veldman PH, Goris R.J. Multiple reflex sympathetic dystrophy. Which patients are at risk for developing a recurrence of reflex sympathetic dystrophy in the same or another limb? Pain 1996 Mar; 64(3):463-466. http://journals.lww.com/pain/Abstract/1996/03000/Multiple_reflex_sym pathetic_dystrophy__Which.8.aspx

4. Maleki J, LeBel AA, Bennett GJ, Schwartzman RJ. Patterns of spread of complex regional pain syndrome, type I (reflex sympathetic dystrophy). Pain 2000; 88: 259-266. https://pubmed.ncbi.nlm.nih.gov/11068113/

5. Kozin F, McCarty DJ, Sims J, et al. The reflex sympathetic dystrophy syndrome. I. Clinical and histologic studies: Evidence of bilaterality, response to corticosteroids and articular involvement. Am J Med 1976; 60:321- 331.
http://www.ncbi.nlm.nih.gov/pubmed/56891?dopt=Abstract

6. Radt P. Bilateral reflex neurovascular dystrophy following a neurosurgical procedure. Clinical picture and therapeutic problems of the syndrome. Confin Neurol 1968; 30:341- 348.
https://www.karger.com/Article/Pdf/103547

7. Hooshmand H, Phillips, EM. Spread of complex regional pain syndrome (CRPS). 2009; 1-11. www.rsdrx.com and www.rsdinfo.com

8.Hooshmand H, Hashmi H. Complex regional pain syndrome (CRPS, RSDS) diagnosis and therapy. A review of 824 patients. Pain Digest 1999; 9:1-24. http://www.rsdrx.com/CRPS_824_Patients_Article.pdf

9. Hooshmand, H, Hashmi, M, Phillips, EM. Cryotherapy can cause permanent nerve damage: A case report. AJPM 2004; 14: 2: 63-70.
http://www.rsdinfo.com/Cryotherapy_Article.pdf

10. Phillips EM. The Misconceptions of complex regional pain syndrome (CRPS). Complex Regional Pain Syndrome (CRPS): Patients' Perspective of Living in Chronic Pain: Volume II. Authors: Alaa ABD-Elsayed and Eric M. Phillips. July 11, 2020.

https://www.amazon.com/gp/product/B08CPBHZP5?ref_=dbs_m_mng_r
wt_calw_tpbk_1&storeType=ebooks

11. Hooshmand H, Phillips EM. Various Complications of Complex
Regional Pain Syndrome (CRPS). Neurological Associates Pain
Management Center, Vero Beach, Florida. www.rsdinfo.com and
www.rsdrx.com Feb 16, 2016.

12. Merskey H, Bogduk N. Classification of Chronic Pain Descriptions of
Chronic Pain Syndromes and Definitions of Pain Terms. Task Force on
Taxonomy of the International Association for the Study of Pain.
Merskey, H. editor. IASP Press. Seattle 1994. http://www.iasp-
pain.org/files/Content/ContentFolders/Publications2/FreeBooks/Classific
ation-ofChronic-Pain.pdf

13. Dielissen PW, Claassen AT, Veldman PH, et al. Amputation for reflex
sympathetic dystrophy. J Bone Joint Surg 1995 ; 77 :270-3.
http://www.ncbi.nlm.nih.gov/pubmed/7706345

14. Veldman PH, Goris RJ. Surgery on extremities with reflex sympathetic
dystrophy. Unfallchirurg 1995; 98:45-48.
http://www.ncbi.nlm.nih.gov/pubmed/7886464

15. Schwartzman RJ, McLellan TL. Reflex sympathetic dystrophy. A
review. Arch Neurol 1987; 44: 555- 561.
http://archneur.jamanetwork.com/article.aspx?articleid=586446

16. Livingston WK. Pain mechanisms: A physiological interpretation of
causalgia and its related states. In London, MacMillan 1944.
https://www.springer.com/gp/book/9781461342946

17. Hooshmand, H, Phillips, EM. Complex regional pain syndrome (CRPS)-Reflex sympathetic dystrophy (RSD) diagnosis and management protocol. 2009. 1-14. www.rsdrx.com and www.rsdinfo.com

18. Veldman PH, Reynen HM, Arntz IE, et al. Signs and symptoms of reflex sympathetic dystrophy: prospective study of 829 patients. Lancet 1993; 342:1012-1016. http://www.ncbi.nlm.nih.gov/pubmed/8105263

19. Cherington M, Happer I, Machanic B, et al. Surgery for thoracic outlet syndrome may be hazardous to your health. Muscle Nerve 1986; 9: 632-634. https://pubmed.ncbi.nlm.nih.gov/3762583/

20. Rowbotham MC. Complex regional pain syndrome type I (reflex sympathetic dystrophy). More than a myth. Editorial. Neurology 1998; 51: 4-5. https://n.neurology.org/content/51/1/4

21. Hooshmand H and Phillips EM. The management of complex regional pain syndrome (CRPS). Neurological Associates Pain Management Center, Vero Beach, Florida. www.rsdinfo.com and www.rsdrx.com Jan 24, 2010.

22. Schwartzman RJ, Erwin KL, et al. "The natural history of complex regional pain syndrome," The Clinical Journal of Pain 2009, Vol. 25, No. 4, 273-280. http://www.ncbi.nlm.nih.gov/pubmed/19590474

23. Hooshmand H, Phillips, EM. Repetitive strain injury (RSI) diagnosis and treatment. 2009; 1-12. www.rsdrx.com and www.rsdinfo.com

24. Schwartzman RJ. Systemic complications of complex regional pain syndrome. Neuroscience & Medicine 2012, 3, 225-242. http://www.scirp.org/journal/PaperInformation.aspx?paperID=22695

25. Rasmussen JW, Grothusen JR, Rosso AL, et al. Atypical Chest Pain: Evidence of Intercostobrachial Nerve Sensitization in Complex Regional Pain Syndrome. Pain Physician 2009; 12: E329-E334. http://www.ncbi.nlm.nih.gov/pubmed/19787018 5

26. Smith JA, Karalis DG, Rosso AL, et al. Syncope in complex regional pain syndrome. Clin Cardiol. 2011 Apr; 34(4):222-225. http://www.ncbi.nlm.nih.gov/pubmed/21462216

27. Benarroch EE. The central autonomic network: functional organization, dysfunction, and perspective. Mayo Clin Proc 1993; 68: 988-1001. http://www.ncbi.nlm.nih.gov/pubmed/8412366

28. Lenz FA, Gracely RH, Zirh AT, et al. The sensory-limbic model of pain memory. Connections from thalamus to the limbic system mediate the learned component of the affective dimension of pain. Pain Forum 1997; 6:22-31. https://www.researchgate.net/publication/257487246_The_sensory-limbic_model_of_pain_memory_Connections_from_thalamus_to_the_li mbic_system_mediate_the_learned_component_of_the_affective_dime nsion_of_pain

29. Gardner FH, Diamond LK. "Autoerythrocyte sensitization; a form of purpura producing painful bruising following autosensitization to red blood cells in certain women," Blood, Vol. 10, No. 7, 1955, 675- 690. http://www.bloodjournal.org/content/bloodjournal/10/7/675.full.pdf

30. Edinger LK, Schwartzman RJ. Gardner-Diamond syndrome associated with complex regional pain syndrome. J Dermatol Case Rep. 2013 Mar 30; 7(1): 10–14. http://www.ncbi.nlm.nih.gov/pmc/articles/PMC3622508/

31. Goris RJA. Skin Complications in RSD. Department of Surgery University Medical Center Nijmegen. Nijmegen 6500 HB, The Netherlands.

32. Galloway NT. Gabale DR, Irwin PP. Interstitial cystitis or reflex sympathetic dystrophy of the bladder? Semin Urol 1991; 9: 148-153. http://www.ncbi.nlm.nih.gov/pubmed/1853012

33. Chancellor MB, Shenot, PJ, Rivas DA, et al. "Urological Symptomatology in Patients with Reflex Sympathetic Dystrophy," Journal of Urology 1996; Vol. 155, No. 2, 634-637. http://www.ncbi.nlm.nih.gov/pubmed/8558679

34. Hooshmand H. RSD Puzzle #127-CRPS and Vulvodynia. http://www.rsdrx.com/RSD_Puzzles_-126- 146.pdf

35. de Klaver MJM, van Rijn MA, Marinus J, et al. Hyperacusis in patients with complex regional pain syndrome related dystonia. J Neurol Neurosurg Psychiatry 2007; 78:1310–1313. https://www.researchgate.net/publication/6360509_Hyperacusis_in_pat ients_with_complex regional_pain_syndrome_related_dystonia

LAURA'S JOURNEY
Laura Vallejos

My first awareness of the disease previously known as reflex sympathetic dystrophy (RSD), but today more familiarly called complex regional pain syndrome (CRPS), was secondhand. Having worked in various healthcare settings as a Unit Coordinator (medical secretary) for three years, and later as a registered respiratory therapist (RRT) for fifteen years, provided opportunities to have worked with patients with this disease. Since I was brought into their care for a heart or lung issue, I did not feel the need to research the disease further. I believed the disease was revealed by its name, one of regional pain, right? Later, I learned first-hand the magnitude of this disease whose name is misleading!

On November 9, 2010, my life abruptly changed before starting my evening shift at the hospital. As, I rounded the corner of the hallway walking towards our department of Cardiopulmonary, my right foot was met by a fast-moving, heavy steel door. It all happened so quickly as the door rode up and lodged midway onto my foot! On the other side of the door was a colleague rushing to an emergency with two oxygen tanks in tow. He was stunned when the door stopped short. Unfortunately, he disregarded the sign on his side of the door which read, "Open door slowly." Once he realized what had occurred, it required both our efforts to free my foot from beneath the door. Despite the immediate pain, I decided to work my shift, hoping the pain would diminish and eventually resolve. I spent my work evening hobbling from one patient room to another with excruciating pain. Although, I considered leaving work early, I felt obligated to stay, since we were already working short staffed.

That first November night as I returned home would be one of many sleepless nights due to the pain, cold and now swollen foot. Upon arriving home from work, I took my routine shower, but I followed it with a hot bath. I was seeking to warm up my noticeably freezing foot. The hot bath did not produce any lasting results since my foot remained extremely cold. As, I attempted to sleep, the weight of the sheet and blankets increased my pain, so I tried to sleep without any covers on my foot. This decision was short lived, since even the air felt too cold for my already freezing foot.

In the morning I reported the incident/injury to my employer's Occupational Health Department. A scheduled appointment with a physician was made and an x-ray was ordered. The results revealed I had suffered a bone contusion, and therefore, I was advised to elevate and ice my foot. A thirty-day supply of Vicodin was prescribed which provided enough relief permitting me to sleep a portion of the night. Since it was determined I did not sustain a fracture, I remained on the work schedule. Almost one month post injury, due to the persistent pain, cold, and swelling, Occupational Health scheduled a Magnetic Resonance Imaging (MRI) scan. The MRI results documented- "extensor hallucis longus tenosynovitis, and changes between the hallux metatarsal head and tibial sesamoid bone. There was also a plantar fibroma and suggestion neuroma between the second and third metatarsophalangeal joints." I received a referral to a Podiatry clinic whose recommendation to be fitted with an arch insert was approved. Although the inserts were made, I never tolerated them and so they went unused.

Void of progress, despite Occupational Health's multiple referrals to specialty physicians, and second opinion consults was discouraging. Although, I continued my forty-hour work week to retain my health benefits, I was in pain daily. Interestingly, the pain changed to a noticeable fire in my foot which strangely moved up my leg and was now noticeably felt in my left foot. Doctor Z-H, provided pain management and prescribed several medications. The gabapentin cream provided no noticeable relief; however, the 5% Lidoderm patch did appear to reduce my pain levels by 10%. I welcomed any amount of reprieve from the pain! Another Podiatrist, Doctor S, was also consulted and he ordered a Triple Phase Bone scan. The scan was not approved by Workman's Compensation and therefore, not performed. Months later, due to the unresolved pain and swelling, I was issued a workability form which allowed me to be off from work for four weeks. During this time, I was instructed to stay off my feet and keep them elevated.

My leisure activities also changed due to my inability to tolerate the pain felt when weight bearing. Prior to my work injury, I spent time walking around the many lakes in Minnesota with friends. Other days, weather permitting, I would bike around the neighborhood for exercise. Consequently, a lack of activity brought an increasing weight gain which did not help an already miserable foot. It took everything in my power to tolerate an eight-hour workday on my feet. Ultimately, I felt I had to choose an eight-hour workday or play? I could no longer tolerate both due to the pain. I chose to work and no longer pursued my leisurely walks.

My symptoms appeared neurological in nature, so I requested Occupational Health to consider approving a consultation with a Neurologist. Unfortunately, my request was denied. Shortly thereafter, my

32

employer scheduled an Independent Medical Examination (IME) to be conducted by Doctor R. Interestingly, Doctor R's, specialty was Neurology. It was this physician who diagnosed my condition two years after my initial injury. He informed me I had "Complex Regional Pain Syndrome (CRPS) which documents as far back as the Civil War." He provided no further details as he hurriedly concluded our session. I was relieved to finally have been given a diagnosis. Once you have a diagnosis, the medical community can implement a plan of action to aid in your recovery. Unfortunately, I was not aware that this disease required a timely diagnosis for a better outcome. At the conclusion of our meeting, I was unaware that this time requirement had already passed.

After receiving the diagnosis of CRPS, I began to research the Twin Cities area for a physician proficient in treating this disease. This inquiry led me to Doctor TH, in St. Paul, Minnesota. Since Worker's Compensation continued my coverage of care, it required their approval. Within a short time, I had received notice permitting me to be treated at this clinic.

During my initial visit with Doctor TH, he was quick to order several treatments and one test. A Nuclear Medicine Three Phase Bone Scan was arranged to assure a fracture was not missed on any previous imaging. Also, a script was issued to begin pool therapy (a pool which has a higher heat content, unlike a traditional heated pool) with a physical therapist. Additionally, a series of lumbar sympathetic blocks were ordered. Doctor TH, also performed a thermal reading on both of my feet after exposing them to the open air for a short time. My right foot had a thermal reading of 26.1 degrees Celsius (78.98 F), while my left foot gave a reading of 28.54 degrees Celsius (83.37 F). Doctor TH, documented, "the right extremity showed signs consistent with CRPS including swelling, temperature

33

changes, discoloration, allodynia, and a global decreased range of motion by 20% of the ankle." Two years post-accident my pain ranged from aching, burning, numbness, and cold. Additionally, I began to experience cramping sensations that originated in my right lower extremity which traveled up affecting my facial muscles.

Not all the requested therapies Doctor TH, ordered were approved at first. Worker's Compensation first denied pool therapy, but later reversed their decision. Eventually, I did complete a total of five lumbar sympathetic blocks administered with I.V. sedation. Although the sympathetic blocks provided immediate results, the pain relief lasted only a day. At the end of the prescribed lumbar injections, I declined any further blocks since they provided no long-term effects. The risks did not outweigh one day of pain relief.

After attending several sessions of pool therapy, the therapy was put on hold after developing an unexplainable, uncontrollable itch, eventually surfacing as a wide-spread rash. I contributed my symptoms to the chlorine in the pool water. Concerned these chemicals may be out of balance, I contacted the facility. After expressing my concerns, the place where I had pool therapy, confirmed and assured me the pool chemicals were not the culprit. After meeting with Doctor TH, to discuss my most recent symptoms, he considered it to be neurodermatitis, a symptom of CRPS. However, he exclaimed since he had never seen neurodermatitis so diffuse in any of his other patients, he provided a Dermatology referral to confirm his suspicions. In the interim, he provided a prescription for Hydroxyzine tablets which were to help in controlling the itch.

Established previously as a patient at the Dermatology clinic, provided a timelier appointment, nevertheless, those few weeks seemed like an eternity. I tirelessly self-medicated with multiple over the counter anti-itch creams and sought alternative remedies such as capsicum capsules. Nothing relieved my symptoms. As I awaited my upcoming appointment with the Dermatologist, I decided to keep my yearly OB-GYN health check-up, despite the rash. Doctor W-H, had been my long-standing gynecologist, who after taking one look at my rash asked, "What the hell happened to you?" Her behavior was not customary; she was always very professional. After explaining my circumstances and upcoming appointment with Dermatology, she insisted on referring me immediately to an Endocrinologist who was able to see me in two days.

Prior to my scheduled appointments, I decided to search the Internet for CRPS organizations. If one existed, I wondered if they could provide me with a remedy I so desperately needed. A quick search provided what would become an invaluable ongoing source of information. I contacted the International RSD Foundation and had an insightful conversation with Mr. Eric Phillips. After explaining my situation to Eric, he suggested an effective treatment plan for the neurodermatitis. He recommended Doxepin Hydrochloride 5% Cream. Now all I needed was a physician who would order the medication!

My awaited appointment with the Endocrinologist arrived, and with me the recommended prescription by Eric. After briefly explaining my health history and recent conversation with the International RSD foundation, the physician did not hesitate to prescribe the Doxepin Cream. This topical cream was highly effective. Immediately upon application it started to subdue the severe itch. The entire tube was almost completely emptied with my first application. The following day I sought a refill, but the pharmacist was reluctant to replenish the supply. However, once the pharmacist contacted the prescribing physician- who stated the rash covered 85% of my body, the prescription was refilled. Within a week, my neurodermatitis was noticeably diminishing, and shortly thereafter, I was able to resume pool therapy.

During one appointment Doctor TH, suggested a ten-week series of acupuncture. These treatments were to be administered by the acupuncturist in his office. I was open to receiving this mode of therapy once approved. I had previously experienced acupuncture one other time in my life, and it went well. My first session with the acupuncturist was barely tolerable, and many of the needles had to be removed due to the pain I was experiencing. She informed me- in the future she would only use the smallest needles obtainable. At a later session, while using the smallest needles she said, "I can actually see your muscles contracting around the needles." I completed the ten-week series hoping to gain advanced wellness, but it never arrived.

Then the unthinkable occurred, another injury to my right foot while at work. The accident occurred while I was in a patient's room performing a tracheostomy dressing change. After removing the soiled dressing and looking to discard it, I was unable to locate the garbage bin. As I searched the room, I noticed it had been placed in the far corner of the room. As I began walking toward the receptacle, I felt a hard jerk on my right ankle. Realizing my foot was caught on something, I found myself hopping on my left foot to avoid an immediate fall. But as my right foot was released, I was propelled forward. I dropped the dirty dressing to break my fall. Unfortunately, as I was falling, I felt the tip of my right tennis shoe catch the floor causing it to hyper plantar flex. Then I heard a loud snap. I found myself on the floor experiencing extreme pain, as my foot began to swell. Coincidentally, the head nurse was passing by the room and saw it all happen. She stopped and said, "That didn't look good! Are you okay?" I replied, "No." She then instructed me to stay down on the floor as she went for a wheelchair and a physician. The long story short- I was diagnosed with a Lisfranc injury (a mid-foot tarsometatarsal fracture).

The new injury brought a heightened exacerbation of my CRPS and a few additional physicians managing my care. Treatment for a Lisfranc injury is usually operative, but instead, I was placed in a removable knee-high boot while the fracture healed. In the days ahead, the intermittent cramping I had previously experienced was now increasingly more severe. The longer I wore the boot, the more severe the cramping. One memorable evening while resting on my back in bed, I began to stretch out my arms and legs. In a flash, my right leg uncontrollably flew away from my body. I thought, "What was that? Well, that is weird!" Baffled by this experience, I was later informed by Doctor TH, I had experienced a flexor spasm. He stated, "Valium will knock it out!" and he ordered Valium to be used as needed. However, Doctor G, a recently consulted physician, prescribed Baclofen to treat the flexor spasms. After completing the first prescription of Valium, I declined any further refills. I believed it did not require two medications to treat the spasms. While employed at my job, I had been exposed to patients struggling with medication addiction. I did not want to take any chances and bring an additional problem into my life. The CRPS was more than enough to contend with.

Since my right foot was extremely sensitive to pressure or any weight resting on it, I asked Doctor TH, if he could order a bed tent for my use.

This device lifts and keeps the bedding off the feet while in bed. I became aware of bed tents while working with patients who underwent various foot surgeries. I was hoping it could possibly allow me to have a more restful and prolonged sleep. Doctor TH, agreed and the tent was ordered. Although I put it to use, the air between the bedding and the mattress felt too cold and became problematic. At first, I tried wearing socks. Unfortunately, the pressure from the socks just irritated my foot and kept me awake. I eventually remedied the situation after purchasing a small, heated foot throw at a local department store which I draped on top of the bed tent. This solution turned out to be ingenious and I was now able to sleep without socks and the air could now be regulated.

I also independently consulted with a dietician (one of the benefits offered by my job), after a blood test ordered by Doctor G, revealed a higher-than-normal level of inflammation in my body. Seeking to reduce this inflammation naturally, a key dietary recommendation was to completely eliminate wheat. The dietician informed me that wheat today is genetically modified (GMO). The GMO wheat triggers an inflammatory response within the body. Thus, I was challenged to keep a wheat free diet for two weeks, and then follow it up by another visit. During this time, I was surprised how much my pain actually decreased once removing this ingredient from my life.

After gaining additional pain relief by eliminating and/or reducing wheat, I decided to seek advice from a Naturopathic physician. Doctor H.H., a Naturopath from St. Paul, Minnesota gave several Homeopathic recommendations after reviewing my medical records. First, after the current value from my Vitamin-D blood test was received, she increased the Vitamin-D3 dosage daily. My results revealed I was sitting at the low end of the normal range and she wanted me to be at the higher end of the normal range. Secondly, a liquid Vitamin-K2 (5 mg.) was prescribed daily for three months, followed by a retest. Thirdly, she prescribed Homeopathic Arnica 200 C daily, to be taken sublingually which she stated was to treat overstrains and old injuries. Fourthly, a prescribed Homeopathic Hypericum (St. John's Wort) was also taken sublingually 2-3 times/day which Doctor HH, stated, "is good for the nerves." Lastly, after providing me with the information, Doctor. HH, encouraged me to consult with a Minnesota Herbalist. I continued on the regimen of supplements she ordered until they were complete. Although I did not experience any noticeable affects during this time, I do not regret her involvement.

The recommended consult by Doctor HH, with the Herbalist rendered immediate and almost complete pain relief! BK, practices as a clinical Herbalist in Winona, Minnesota. At the end of my visit, she prepared and applied a topical herbal poultice which she secured to the top of my right foot. To release the herbal medicinal properties, a small amount of olive oil was poured over the dry herbs contained in this pouch. My foot was then wrapped in a plastic bag which helped contain the oil and herbs as it leaked out over the foot. I was instructed to wear this for several days, and at the end of that time, to call the clinic with an update on my condition. Although it remained a messy application, within hours, my foot pain was barely noticeable! As instructed, I contacted BK, with the amazing results, and she mailed out additional poultices for my future use. However, due to the difficulty in wearing and keeping a weeping poultice in place could not justify its continuous or long-term use.

A conflict in care eventually arose when two separate physicians involved in my recovery had opposing treatment plans. An attempt to increase my current four-hour workday, limited due to symptoms, Doctor G, ordered a rolling knee walker. I was instructed to use this device while at work and at home. I noticed the longer I used the rolling knee walker, my spasms became more frequent, and my pain heightened. Fortunately, it was during this time when a purchased book recommended by Eric from the International RSD Foundation had arrived in the mail. Doctor Hooshmand's book, "Chronic Pain Reflex Sympathetic Dystrophy Prevention and Management" could not have arrived in a timelier fashion. As I read through the material it revealed many of my symptoms. Doctor Hooshmand's research attributes too much activity, or too little can worsen CRPS symptoms. Since, I was experiencing escalating symptoms, I contributed it to the constant use of this device. In contrast, Doctor TH, encouraged me to join a health club and continue pool therapy (a non-weight bearing activity) now that both land and pool therapy were complete. He wrote an order for me to join a health club that housed a therapy pool on their premise and encouraged my attendance at least three times a week. The initial joining fee and membership for six months was paid for by Worker's Compensation.

Once the prescribed therapies were completed with little advancement, my employer decided I could no longer do my job. I was asked to attend a scheduled meeting with Human Resources. I was told I had been a great employee, but they had to let me go since I could not tolerate being on my feet for any sufficient length of time. Near the end of the meeting, the Occupational Health nurse stated, "If you can ever get back on your feet again, you can come back, and your boss would hire you again immediately."

After my job loss, a few things changed. I completely abandoned the restricting rolling knee walker, but continued pool therapy diligently. One year later, I had increased this non-weight bearing exercise to an hour without increasing my symptoms. Also, the medication Baclofen was discontinued and replaced with an over-the-counter oral supplement containing MHB3 Hyaluronan. I became aware of the supplement Hyaluronan while attending the Fourth International Fascia Research Congress in Reston, Virginia in 2015. Doctor PR, a physician-scientist and Director of the Motor Recovery Research Laboratory at the New York Rusk Institute of Rehabilitation Medicine was a presenting lecturer. Her presentation documented the results of a series of injections of Hyaluronan (non-FDA approved at that time) administered to a patient she had met two-years post stroke. The patient had suffered a complete paralysis of their right hand and arm which was tightly contracted. The results from the injected Hyaluronan, documented via video, provided astonishing results. After completing three series of injections several weeks apart, this man was able to demonstrate complete voluntary movement of his right hand. Everyone attending this lecture were amazed. I also was astounded by this neurological research. Although my neurological injury was peripheral, I questioned if additional recovery could be attained with Hyaluronan. I verbally stated out loud, "I need that stuff!" A physician sitting beside me replied, "You can get that stuff, but not by injection." When the lecture concluded, the physician sitting beside me gave me information on an oral Hyaluronan (Baxyl) that could be purchased online. After arriving home from the conference, I ordered my first bottle. Within a week the cramping lessened. As I continued taking this product my cramping and flexor spasms disappeared completely, so I

41

quit taking the Baclofen. A milestone was reached that day, one of increasing recovery!

Twelve-years, have now passed since my first injury, and though I hope for a remission, it has not arrived. I am vigilant and continue to maintain my progress. Today, my exercise regimen continues and may even include a leisurely thirty-minute walk. Although the neurodermatitis occasionally flares, it is no longer widespread and does resolve after applying the Doxepin cream. The pain in the foot is constant, but waxes and wanes due to my activity, and Minnesota weather. I continue to treat my pain with a Lidoderm patch or cream as needed. Additionally, after being approved to the MinnMed program in Minnesota, I have the option to apply a topical cream containing cannabidiol and/or tetrahydrocannabinol (CBD/THC). This cream has provided additional pain relief when the Lidoderm is not sufficient. The bed tent and heated foot throw remain a permanent fixture on my bed and still provide relief to my still freezing foot. Also, by reducing wheat from my diet, although difficult (since wheat is an ingredient in many products), it has allowed me to keep my pain levels down. Today, I prefer to wear sandals when the weather permits, otherwise, I tolerate only loose-fitting socks and a larger shoe size. My preinjury shoe size was 8.5, but today I require a 10 WW shoe/boot which can accommodate my right foot when it swells.

If you, or someone you know, have been diagnosed with this disease, I hope the information I have shared is useful as we wait for the medical community to make advancements. May our future bring with it a remission and/or a complete healing.

PROCEDURE FROM HELL: MY CRPS STORY
Anonymous

To tell my story, I must first start with my past. When I was a toddler about three-years-old, I was told I was raped by a teenage boy. Then at the ages of five and six, I was sexual abused by my mother's boyfriend, who was also a police officer. He physically abused my mother and sexually abused both me and my sister. My sister received the brunt of it as she was trying to protect me even at that young age (she is only 15-months older than me). I had blocked this out until I was an adult in my 30s.

We'll come back to my past in a second, now fast forward to the future. I have had back problems since my 20s. After multiple Rhizotomies, I eventually had a 360° fusion, which fixed my back. I then reinjured my back working for the school system; I taught three to five-year-old special needs students for nine years. This was now a worker's comp case. I could not switch doctors until my case was settled. But I trusted my doctor, why would I change?

After reinjuring my back my pain management doctor recommended, I have a spinal cord stimulator (SCS) implanted. I agreed and we scheduled the trial SCS for February 2018. During the procedure, the doctor only gave me valium to put me to sleep. Although, I do not remember the actual procedure, I was awakened with an extremely sore throat after the procedure. I asked a tech why my throat hurt so badly? I was told that I screamed throughout the entire procedure. The doctor actually came in and apologized for the procedure. That would be the only apology I would receive from her. I woke up not only with a sore throat, but my body from the waist down was on fire, jumpy, felt like electric shocks coursing through my legs, and it felt like millions of red ants biting me. My fusion was not nearly as painful as this, and I was cut open in my stomach and my back for that surgery. I walked into that building with some pain, I was wheeled out in excruciating pain, and I was unable to walk.

A SCS has two leads for each side of the spine. My doctor was able to get the first lead positioned, however the second lead gave her trouble. She put the second lead in and then pulled it back out because it would not go all the way in properly. She tried to repositioned the one lead to hit both sides of my spine. She also cut too high on my spine for the SCS. I was told I could meet with the tech if I needed to lower or raise the pulses from the SCS. I met with him the next day and asked him to turn it off. I was in AGONY!

For my follow up appointment, I had to show up using a walker. I was dragging my left leg behind me, and my pain level was a 10/10. She removed the lead and proceeded to diagnose me with Conversion Disorder. I was told my pain was not real. She prescribed me Vicodin as she diagnosed me with a disorder that said my pain was not real. Her reasoning behind her diagnosis was from the trauma I went through as a child. She actually covered up what she did by blaming the abuse I received as a child was the reasoning behind my pain. What makes it worse, she did not tell me about this new diagnosis. I discovered it six-months later when I ordered my medical records and read it for myself. I ordered my medical records because my tests kept getting denied, due to her diagnosis of conversion disorder. But I still received my pain medications every month without fail. I had gone to my neurosurgeon and he order the same tests and they were approved. Why? Because he did not have a diagnosis of

Conversion Disorder attached to his records. This wasted six months of my life, because she did not come clean about what she had done. It was then I learned I had to be my own advocate. It was a hard lesson to learn.

Now back to my past. I began having dreams of the abuse. I asked my sister and she said yes, it was true. I was broken. I happened to have had an appointment with my doctor not long after these dreams. I trusted her, because she was my doctor. I told her what had happened to me as a child. Little did I know that she would use this against me in the future to diagnose me with Conversion Disorder.

My doctor was on vacation, so I had to see her partner. By this point I had had an EMG that proved I had some sort of nerve damage in my spine. Proving that my pain was indeed real. I told this doctor everything. Everything that is written above I told him. He apologized profusely, and he made an amendment to my medical record showing I did not have Conversion Disorder, and he took over my treatment.

The following month when I went for my appointment. My old doctor did not work there any longer. Fast forward a few more months, I was able to settle my workers' comp case and I found a new doctor, Doctor NH, my hero. On my first visit he had me diagnosed with complex regional pain syndrome (CRPS). Due to my epilepsy, I cannot take nerve pain medication. They make my seizures worse. I have tried a few different ones with the same result. So, the only thing I can take is pain medications. After, years of being on low dose Vicodin, it had taken its toll. I was depressed. Doctor NH, switched me from Vicodin to Percocet and that helped tremendously. The suicide thoughts had stopped. I am prescribed 10 mg of Percocet twice a day. I also take Magnesium (for pain), Turmeric (for pain), Ashwagandha (for anxiety) supplements. I have had 10 sympathetic nerve blocks so far, and currently have two more scheduled.

My CRPS has spread from my left foot and calf to the right foot, and I am currently starting to get tingles and aching in my left knee. Due to using a cane and putting too much weight on my right side, I have developed arthritis in my right elbow and right hip. I recently had a platelet-rich plasma (PRP) procedure in my hip and elbow, which was extremely painful and is currently not covered by insurance. The procedure cost is $700. The easiest way to explain this is they take a big tube of my blood, clean it to get the plasma and then reinject the plasma into the joint. It is supposed to help regenerate the cells and lead to healing. The jury is still out on whether or not it worked. Although my hip does not burn as much as it did before the PRP procedure. Not sure about the elbow as of yet.

I now have a boot, a walker, a wheelchair, and a cane that I use for flare ups. The boot, wheelchair, and walker are new due to the intensity of my flare ups. My extreme moments of pain can last from a few hours, to a few days, or for a few weeks. They have gotten much worse, more intense, and more often. I had not used the walker since my original diagnosis in 2018.

I had to borrowed a walker from my grandmother. I am 44-years-old, handicapped, deal with intense pain daily. I also currently work a 40-hour week at a hospital. I am a certified patient access representative for insurance verification. I volunteered to work in the ER when my department shut down due to Covid. I now would not be able to do that because I am unable to push the computer around going from room to room to register patients. This disorder has taken my pride, my self-confidence, my self-reliance. I have to depend on my husband, and my children. It's sad that my children have to see me like this and worry about me all the time. This is what hurts me the most. I have missed out on birthday parties, family gatherings, trips all because of this disorder, but I have learned to live with this. I have learned to live with the pain, the stares, the judgement I see from extended family and others. CRPS is something I have, and although it tries, it will NOT define me. I am so much stronger than CRPS.

A MOTOR BIKE RIDE THAT TURNED INTO CRPS
Kelly Cielanga

My complex regional pain syndrome (CRPS) started on August 10, 2013, after a motor bike accident where I was thrown from the back seat, I hit the ground and I slid about 12-feet on the ground. I had several breaks. I broke my scapula, four ribs, a finger and my left foot.

The Insurance Corporation of British Columbia (ICBC), made me do physical therapy right after the boot came off. My foot had not healed, so after several visits to a podiatrist, he sent me to a specialist who sent me for several test to confirm I had complex regional pain syndrome (CRPS), so it would be recognized by ICBC, and that my lawyer could fight for compensation. It took me eight months to get my official diagnosis of CRPS.

This is where the real battle began. I was then put through a slew of physical test by ICBC to prove I was disabled even though the test said I had CRPS. I was also made to do a few sympathetic nerve blocks, the ones you where have to lay on your stomach and they inject anesthesia and steroids into the sympathetic nerve along-side your spinal cord. Needless to say, it did not work, and not to mention the crazy number of drugs you are made to try that result in mood swings, depression, and huge weight gain.

So, for four-years, I had to jumped threw the ICBC hoops to qualify for disability. I could no longer work with the pain levels and the limited mobility of my foot.

After settling, ICBC started taking control of my treatment and drug prescriptions which I have to say nothing works for me other than a low dose of naltrexone.

I do have an awesome pain specialist but he is learning along with me about this disease. After six-years I am now full body affected. One of my worst experiences was thinking I was having a heart attack, and having my youngest son take me into emergency sitting down with the intake nurse telling her my symptoms and also saying I had CRPS.

After that I sat in waiting room for 20-minutes scarred out of my mind but trying not to worry my son. I was then taken into emergency room and treated like I was a chronic pill seeker. I started doing research on my own. CRPS can affect the internal organs but most doctors in my world do not recognize this, so now I have a fear of not being listened to. So, I just ride out any internal issues right now I am battling with my new doctor over high blood pressure, high cholesterol, high blood sugars and being able to lose weight.

Until, I can find someone that can treat it as part of the effects of CRPS I am afraid I will never make headway on any issues, until a doctor realizes you have to treat all of the issues not just the single ones, and pills are not always the answer.

CPRS: BY THE HANDS OF SOMEONE ELSE
Marilyn Roth

My story begins with a Trigger finger surgery on April 20, 2018. I went in for a simple procedure and woke up in a cast up to my elbow. I could not understand what was happening. The pain was unbearable after surgery. I had to take dilaudid for the pain.

I am a 2005 Cancer survivor so I know what pain is. At that time, I had my uterus removed. I never had any kind of pain like this. I also suffer from degenerative disc disease which I had been on pain medications prior.

After a few days I quickly realized brain fog , and burning-hot/ice-cold uncontrollable pain. I knew something was not right. Once the cast came off after 10-days my fingers would not move, and they curled under and became stiff. I then went to see a hand specialist who said the word complex regional pain syndrome (CRPS), which I had never heard of before. The doctor I was seeing ordered me to have a three-phase bone scan at that time. To complicate the situation, I had then received a notice from the medical board stating that the doctor performed the surgery at the wrong site (area), it was now the end of October 2018.

So instead of trigger finger surgery they had performed a wrist surgery of some kind, and to this day it is unclear what surgery was done. I now suffer from headache, tremors, PTSD ,mood swings, sensitivity to anything that touches my hand, or fingers. My hand gets hot, cold, turns purple, and I lost all function in the right hand and fingers. The bone scan showed decrease blood flow consistent with CRPS. Physical therapy was ordered but it was so painful and my bones were now fused in that position.

A year ago, I was seen by Doctor in Los Angeles, CA who is the top CRPS Doctor. He confirmed it was CRPS after extensive testing. A few weeks ago, I returned to see this Doctor and the temperature has decreased by three degrees lower in my hand and fingers and it is 30% worse all together. The CRPS has now spread into my left side of my neck and my outcome does not look good.

I have taken a class for the spinal cord stimulator (SCS),but due to other things like degenerative disc and stenosis it may not be a good thing. Due to the outstanding litigation, it has prolonged my treatment I am now looking at ketamine treatment for the future. It has been a journey my life is forever changed like so many of us who suffer from this disease. I pray for a cure to come and for those Doctors who come in contact with CRPS patients to be compassionate and kind. I want doctors to please listen to our concerns.

Thank you for allowing me to tell my story.

HOW MY LIFE CHANGED
Karen Crabb

My Complex regional pain syndrome (CRPS) started when I had my accident in June 2016. I stood on a lose paving slab on a farm that my husband and I were renting. I had just come home from my shift as an **Accident and Emergency Nurse** and said to my husband I was going to the top of the garden to check on my vegetables that I was growing.

It was a beautiful sunny day, so I went up the steps and checked my vegetables. There was one paving slab that had been put there (not by us) but, little did I know this paving slab was not placed properly. I stood on it, and I felt it moving, so I tried to balance myself as it moved.

Unfortunately, the paving slab won and I went over. I tried to save myself with my right foot as I landed on my left side. I saw the bone in my right ankle snap and push my skin out. I screamed and my husband heard me, he ran out and knew straight away it was broken. He called for an ambulance and unfortunately, living on a farm, it took three hours for the Paramedics to find it.

So, I laid outside in agony, until they eventually arrived. Then it started to rain, and they were trying to sedate me. It was not fun and the pain was getting worse. The next day I was operated on, I had eight pins, a plate and two bolts placed in my ankle on the left side and right side.

After my operation, I was in the ward, and my surgeon came to see me and he told me, unfortunately, during the operation my peripheral nerve was damaged, and they tried to find it to repair it but, he could not repair it.

I was not weight bearing for seven-weeks with leg in a cast. I started to suffer pain while having the cast on. The pain was so intense at the back of my heel I had the urge to have my cast removed thinking that it was the pressure from it causing this tremendous pain, it was such a very sharp intense digging pain. I even went to hospital to tell them, but nothing was done.

After my cast was finally removed, my mobility was so poor, so I struggled a lot. I started with physio therapy. I was in physio therapy for over a year. All this time I was telling them about the burning sensation I was getting, the swelling I had and my foot was turning a purple color, and the pain was so intense.

I was told that because of the metal in my ankle, the swelling will be the reason this was happening and it will ease soon. I still have a lot of intense jerks in my foot they are so force-full that it sets the pain off worse. The pins and needles and burning, and the cold and hot sensations are just too much to handle.

Things only got worse. I remember I started to get a strange sensation that something wet was on my ankle but it was dry to the touch. I also had the feeling of a cold breeze blowing on my foot. In October 2016, I developed a deep vein thrombosis (DVT) in my right calf, so I was put on blood thinners for three months.

So many times, I visited my general practitioner (GP) and told him all the symptoms I was having. Eventually, I was sent to a Neurologist in September 2017, and I was finally diagnosed with complex regional pain syndrome (CRPS)-Type II.

At this point my mobility was getting effected. I was using a walking stick and a mobility scooter when I went out. The stairs were a big problem, so eventually, we had to leave the farm and move to a Bungalow.

Treatment

I tried so many medications to try to control my pain, and my depression. At this time, I could no longer work as a nurse. I was no longer able to wear shoes that covered my foot, because the sensation of anything touching it would cause it to swell, and set the pain off.

On a scale of 0 to 10 the only ease I got was keeping my foot elevated, so it was not touching the ground, and to this day I still have to do this to help with the swelling, and the color changes.

When I saw my specialist, I mentioned the issue I was having with my foot. I was told anything that touches my foot, was because the nerve that was damaged became aggravated and that the swelling will never go away.

I had two nerve blocks in my ankle and it made my condition worse. Now am still on controlled drugs, and awaiting now to see a neurosurgeon to talk about having a spinal cord stimulator (SCS) fitted.

In May 2020, I started to get symptoms of CRPS in my right foot. I have developed burning pain, spasms, and a cold breeze feeling blowing in my foot. I had mentioned this to my pain consultant. He had said that CRPS can spread to your opposite limb.

At the present time the doctor is investigating this, and I am waiting for the outcome. I have seen an orthopaedic doctor and recently had an MRI, on the 18th of this month I will know if there is something else going on with my left foot, before my pain consultant can confirm that my CRPS has spread.

I have found with this condition it not only affects my mobility, my mood , but I seem to suffer now with gastric issues, and anxiety. My hair, my nails have all changed. My nails seem to have stopped growing, my hair is so dry it's like straw, and clumps up . I have gained weight , from my medication but also the CRPS and lack of mobility, and not being able to do any exercises.

Water is an issue for me , long gone the days I could have a soak in a bath, now it's a quick shower, and that's because the water feels like pins hitting my foot .

Sleep, I can go to bed, but I am back up within an hour, due to pain and the intense jerks I suffer from. This causes me to be up for hours. Also, the sheets touching my foot causes me more pain.

I now claim disability for mobility and have adaptations to be able to drive my car with my left foot, which is an automatic car.

This is going to be reviewed as now driving with my left foot my toes and the symptoms of CRPS in my left foot is having an effect now. My memory is terrible, I suffer with a lot of brain fog.

I have taken up Art, to distract me from the pain I suffer from. So, when my mood allows me, I do acrylic painting, and I also enjoy listening to music.

My husband and family (as in my children) who live away from me sort of understand, but I tend not to mention my pain or my symptoms because I feel they are fed-up of it now.

It is so unfortunate, that the NHS here in England are not aware of CRPS. So, most visits to hospital you have to explain the condition to them. As a nurse myself, I had never heard of CRPS, and I feel this is where others such as family, friends, and the public do not understand or they feel that people who suffer from CRPS just exaggerate about what they go through. This is because there is not awareness about the condition.

I always feel that we are left on a shelf to get on with this, and where I live in South Wales, the health board here does not offer the same treatment as the rest of England does .

I joined a few CRPS groups on Facebook to be able to talk to others who suffer from CRPS, to share my concerns, and get some advice.

THE UNEXPECTED JOURNEY OF LIFE
Kayla S.

In, January 2017, I had just turned 24-years-old. I was working at my first full-time job since graduating college. I was running half marathons, playing volleyball, working with dogs, and exploring my backyard mountains. I was working at a wastewater facility at the time. Ice is notorious for forming on all surfaces at the facility. I just walked out of our disinfection building, assuming all the walkways had been salted, and my life changed. I rolled my foot hard. Shortly after, I had stabbing pain in the middle of my foot. I was examined at urgent care that day. They could not find anything wrong and sent me home with a boot, which was oversized. Over the course of the next 12-months, I saw numerous doctors, physical therapists, and orthopedic specialists. Not one could see why I had pain.

Twelve months after the initial injury, I saw a new doctor in the new town I moved to. Immediately, Doctor G, saw I had a fracture that never healed. After another six months of trying to heal it naturally, in June 2018, I finally had the first midfoot fusion to correct it. It took a long time to heal. Even after a year of exercise and physical therapy, I still had muscle spasms and could not go further than four miles. Flash forward to November of 2019. The sharp stabbing pain came back. I saw Doctor G, again who found a fracture next to the original break that was damaged due to the weight shift in the foot bones. We tried a bone stimulator and other various things to remedy the fracture. Surgery was suggested after four months of nothing working.

COVID hit, which delayed the next midfoot fusion surgery, until September 2020. At this point, my mental health was suffering. I had gained 70 pounds since I broke my foot. I already feared this surgery would not work after the first one failed. I grieved the loss of my mobility. I got out of surgery early and Doctor G, said it went beautifully. He used less hardware and got the foot cleaned up from the buildup from the first surgery. I was feeling confident. Week eight of non-weight bearing was up and I still felt like surgery was that morning.

The pain never stopped. The incision was not healing; Doctor G, had repeatedly debrided it to try to stimulate healing. Shoes were excruciating to wear and I would feel like puking when I put the compression socks on. I was referred to a physical therapist that was going to help me try to regain my strength. J, is an incredible therapist. We tried lasers, needling, and other more complicated physical therapy to get my foot healing. We did this for six weeks and it got worse every week. By this time, I had been seeing a psychologist for about a year and still to this day. My psychologist did cognitive behavioral therapy, mindfulness practice, and eye movement desensitization and reprocessing (EMDR) to help me out.

At the end of December 2020, I saw Doctor G, again. He was disappointed that it was only getting worse. At this point he touches my foot to test the pain level. I burst into tears. He then stated that I developed complex regional pain syndrome (CRPS). The pain was life altering and only got worse each week. A soft breeze of air felt like razor blades were being dragged across the top of my foot. Socks felt like an elephant was crushing my foot. My foot got stiff like a board and felt cold like it was put into a freezer all day. My foot would spasm constantly. My skin, muscles, and bones started to deteriorate. I kept seeing J, for physical therapy each week. We tried to do graded motor imagery and mirror therapy with it. Doctor G, referred me to a pain management specialist across the road. This specialist is young. Doctor C, said this was CRPS and he could help. Early-January 2021, Doctor C, performed a spinal nerve block. During the procedure I was becoming more and more in pain. I explained I was in so much pain not just in my foot, but now is my back, hip, and leg. He left the room explaining to me that it would take a day or so to feel better. Well, 24-hours later, I was physically unable to walk due to the extreme pain. I went to the ER where they gave me some sleep aids and pain medication. They sent me on my way since the botched nerve block would just take some time to heal.

The end of January, all of February, and into March 2021, are a complete blur. After, I had this horrifying nerve block, Doctor G, put me on Lyrica and combined it with Cymbalta. We tried all the combinations and I have no idea what happened. I remember being in so much pain one day that I just stopped taking all the medications. I then came out of the terrible medicine fog. I was in so much pain every day. I wanted it all to end. There were many moments I thought about cutting my own leg off and had a couple instances of suicidal ideations. It was the darkest moments of my life.

March 2021, I started seeing Doctor E, who was supposed to be the best for CRPS. He tried two more spinal nerve blocks, which at best gave me 50% relief for just shy of 24-hours. Each procedure I would have a panic attack because I knew the pain would only get worse if it did not work. He was valiant in his efforts to help. May 2021, we had finished the blocks and were prepping to do a spinal cord stimulator (SCS). The large possibility of having treatment resistant CRPS was looming overhead. Each procedure made the CRPS worse. I was losing my ability to walk entirely. I was walking with a cane and a knee crutch every day.

With nothing giving me any relief, I started delving into non-traditional ways to heal. I tried Reiki energy healing, witchcraft, herbalism, Chinese medicines and herbs, pulsed electromagnetic field therapy (PEMF) machines, and many other non-traditional methods. The Reiki energy healing helped me mentally the most. It helped me grieve the loss of my leg while giving me a few good days of sleep.

By the end of July 2021, we got the trial for the SCS in. The surgery was difficult and painful. The device was placed but there was no relief. After three days of trying the SCS, we had to reprogram it due to no relief. The rest of the trial, I spent with no relief. I saw Doctor E, at the beginning of August 2021 to remove the SCS trial. I asked what more we could do, knowing full well there were not many options left. He suggested I meet Doctor B, a neurosurgeon, and Doctor H, an orthopedic surgeon who has performed CRPS amputations.

I met Doctor H, first. He had explained he had done several amputations that were successful in CRPS patients. He said the only other thing we could try is have Doctor B, perform a peripheral nerve stimulator before amputation. I met with Doctor B, who is world renowned. Doctor B, tried to tell me about this stimulator and that it might help, but since I had doubts due to the SCS failing, he did not feel confident to proceed with the stimulator. We scheduled the amputation.

With the amputation set, it was time to prepare myself. I spoke to several people who were CRPS amputees in very similar situations. I spoke to many amputees as well. Each one had a unique outcome, but not one regretted the decision. It was a 50/50 shot to work. I was no longer physically able to walk. On one hand we had a good chance for success, on the other hand held a more difficult outcome. If it were to work, I would likely have phantom pain. The terrible trade off being that phantom pains come and go while the CRPS pain is 24/7. I weighed my options and decided this hail Mary was a better chance to regain mobility.

September 30, 2021, is a day I soon will not forget. Amputation day! Since the SCS trial, I only slept one to four hours a night. My body was rejecting food. I lost 20 pounds in a month. To say I was on my last leg was truly accurate. We arrived at the hospital. They took several tries, but got the IV in finally. There was no sense of panic or doubt in the air. I had my team of doctors to help me. We were ready. They took me to the operating room, placed the epidural, and put me to sleep.

I almost instantaneously sat up once the medication wore off. I sat up in a bolt because there was no pain. No muscle spasms. No freezing cold foot. I was free. I cried tears of joy. Doctor H, came to check on me, and I told him I felt like I could run a half marathon. Each day, I got better. Stronger. Happier. I got discharged on day four, after hopping down the hall and back with a huge smile on my face. I am sleeping seven to eight hours a night again. I am able to eat food again. I am pain free. As I write this, I feel grateful that I found a solution to the pain. I beat CRPS. It has only been two weeks after my surgery and what tiny amounts of phantom sensations/pain has been so miniscule and been for just a couple minutes. I have been nearly pain-free every day since the amputation. I never thought my life would go down this path, but I know that if I can handle CRPS, I can handle anything.

Thank you, to everyone who provided knowledge, and experience about CRPS and amputation. I cannot thank each one of you enough. Without hearing your stories, I may never have considered amputation. I am thankful for the team of doctors who were kind and helpful along my journey.

"HOPE"
Ginger Osness

I was a healthy 33-year-old. I had no health problems, just a minor allergy to Penicillin. It was a nice spring night in May of 2016. My son was in his freshmen year, and had a baseball double header in our local town. He was pitching. The whole family came out to watch. It was such a wonderful evening. My nieces and nephews running around the park, proud parents and grandparents watched on. After the game, clumsy me, I tripped and fell. I had instant pain to my left pinkie finger. When I had the courage to look at it, I realized that it was dislocated. In the ED, the finger was set the best it could be, and I was told to follow up with a specialist on Monday, because the finger was also fractured.

So, Monday came, and in my consult, I was told I would need a minor surgery and a pin to be placed to hold the finger and fracture in place to heal. The pin was to be in place for five weeks. By Wednesday, I went in for surgery. I was terrified, but made it through.

After surgery, my husband was home to care for me. I kept on top of my pain medications, but my pain was always so much more at night, which is not uncommon after surgery. About a week had passed, and I started to experience severe burning pain to my hand. No way to cool it off, as it was wrapped up, and the wrap was not to be removed. I requested a refill on my Vicodin to no avail. The nurse treated me rudely as if I were drug seeking, and told me I should not be having that much pain anymore. I had about five Vicodin left, and started to ration what I had left, and only took enough to take the edge off, splitting my medication in halves. Night after night, the burning kept me up at night, I would lay in bed and cry. I went back a couple of times demanding to be seen. They re-wrapped my hand multiple times, thinking the wrap and position of my wrist maybe needed to be adjust. It did not help. I remember calling the surgeon begging her to remove the pin. Eventually, week five came, and she removed the pin. It hurt, but I felt almost instant relief!! Finally, I thought, this nightmare is over!! Little did I know what was going to lie ahead.

I started occupational therapy (OT) to get my finger moving again, as it was very stiff. We worked and worked to try to get my finger to bend and or move. Minimal movement. I remember the OT hand therapist getting frustrated and saying "now just pick up this cup and wrap your finger around it." I could not do it no matter how hard I tried. Weeks had gone by, it remained swollen. I would sit for hours doing my exercises trying to get the joints in my finger to move. I remember lying in bed one night, in extreme pain, not being able to sleep. Suddenly, my finger literally started to drip sweat. Just that finger. It was incredibly scary; it was so weird. What the heck was going on.

One Saturday afternoon, I met a nurse practitioner out and about, who looked at my swollen blue hand, and said very bluntly to me, "you have complex regional pain syndrome (CRPS)." I did not know what to think, I am a nurse, and I had never learned this from my college education, nor had I ever heard of it. I went home and of course did a little doctor google, I was shocked. Of course, this is what I had. The color changes, swelling, pain, burning, sweating, all the symptoms matched.

Back to the doctor that Monday, as I watched my hand turn blue and purple and red all weekend. It would sweat and sweat and get so very hot.

I waited in the doctor's office for the surgeon to come in. She walked in and I started to cry. She took one look at my hand and said, it looks like you may have CRPS. The ortho surgeon spent an hour with me, consoling me, and wrote me for an urgent referral to the pain clinic in her building. This is where things took a bad turn for me.

The pain doctor, Doctor R, saw me within two days. He did a full exam, and was not convinced it was CRPS. I went over all of my symptoms, including the pain. He saw the color changes and sweating. He started me on Gabapentin just in case and some topicals. The gabapentin was to be increased slowly until the pain was relieved. The pain continued to get worse, and I was having extreme anxiety. Doctor R, would not diagnose me with CRPS. He was not ready to do a nerve block. One visit, he said to me " It can't possibly be CRPS if you have no pain. You are acting crazy." I started to cry, and continued to tell him it was burning. I left in tears. He was not listening to me, and I felt defeated. My doctor thinks I am crazy, and I started to feel like I was headed down that path. The more I increased the gabapentin, the worse I felt. I was not sleeping or eating. The pain was getting worse, not better, and the symptoms started to spread all the way up my arm.

Finally, I got a second opinion. Doctor F, was my healthcare knight in shining armor. There I was, sobbing in his office, which I could tell made him uncomfortable. He is not the kind of doctor that does not want to see people suffer, I was suffering. He took one look at my hand, and finally gave me a diagnosis of CRPS. He scheduled nerve blocks, counseling, and therapy. Unfortunately, I continued to get worse. I was only sleeping about three hours a night, I was not eating, and the 1800mg of gabapentin was not helping. I remember calling a friend one Saturday morning, because I was going crazy. I wanted to get help and commit myself, but I knew that I would not get pain relief in a place like that. So, what other option did I have. I had lost 25 pounds from my 5'2" frame in two months, was always on flight or fight not sleeping. I was done. I did not want to live the rest of my life like this. She talked me down, and told me to reach out to my doctor. Now as a nurse, I should have known to do this, but when you are in so much pain, anxiety, no sleep, no eating, your mind does not seem to work as well as it should. I saw my doctor and got on Effexor, Trazodone, Ambien, and a short-term RX for Xanax. It helped, but I still could not sleep, and this continued my vicious cycle of pain. I would show up to the pain clinic every week unannounced desperate for someone to take my pain away. There had to be something they could do. Doctor F, gave me a prescription for Nucynta. My counselor in the meantime suggested to Doctor F, that I get off the Gabapentin. I did and started Lyrica. My medication regimen now consisted of Effexor, trazadone, Xanax, Ambien, Lyrica, Voltaren gel, Lidocaine gel, Nucynta, Flexeril, Vitamin C, Alpha Lipoic Acid, and who knows what other vitamins. After the Gabapentin was out of my system, I started to sleep. Sleep is an amazing thing. It is one thing I will never take for granted again. Going to bed early and naps I will never apologize for or fight.

I spent a good six months in a constant cycle of flight or fight, making my situation worse. Would sit at my desk crying, obsessed about my hand. It is hard not to do, when it hurts all the time. I almost lost my job. My marriage suffered and I almost lost my husband as well. There is no way, if I would not have gotten my anxiety state more in control, that he would have been able to handle being married to me forever.

After seven nerve blocks, numerous medications, a drug study in Madison, WI, acupressure, acupuncture, massage, years of PT and OT, and pain psychology, things finally got better. Pain psychology and not letting the pain control my life was the biggest help. I do believe though that it was a multi-disciplinary process. Each therapy helped me in some way or another…. Except the acupuncture. That was a definite ouch. Once I was able to just deal with the pain and keep moving in my life, I felt better more and more. It took years though.

I was able to wean off all of my medications except for my as needed pain medication. I still will have flares that last a few days, but for the most part my pain has considerably decreased.

It took years, but I wanted to share my story, because there is hope. I crawled out of the darkest place in my life both medically, physically, and emotionally. Do not give up, keep going. The more I accepted my life with pain, and the more I did not let it stop me from living my life, the better life got.

I know that I have to be careful, so sports is a no go for me anymore. I stick to walking and swimming for exercise. And of course, I could not have done it without my faith in Jesus. I learned to stop thinking how this disease wrecked me, and started to Thank the Lord that I am able to live a normal life again, even with pain. He truly has blessed me.

THE MONSTER WITHIN:
MY STORY OF VENIPUNCTURE CRPS
Amy S.

My story with complex regional pain syndrome (CRPS), began on June 4, 2001. That morning I woke up, and it felt like any other day. Later during the morning, I started feeling a fullness type of pain in my chest. At first, it was not too painful, but the pain seemed to worsen as the day went on. I took an over-the-counter pain reliever to alleviate the pain, but it did not help. The pain became worse, finally later in the afternoon I sought medical attention since the pain had not been helped by pain relievers. So, I decided to go to an urgent care facility, once I was there, I was taken to an examining room and assessed by a medical assistant, soon after a doctor came in and examined me. He decided to have my chest and abdomen X-rayed, and have some blood-work taken. A medical assistant came in and attempted to draw my blood through a needle stick, she turned my wrist to the side and decided to stick the needle in through the side of my wrist, at that moment when the needle went in I felt an intensive sharp pain, I told her that something was wrong, this was not like a normal blood draw that I have experienced in the past, she assured me it was fine, but I noticed no blood was entering the vial, she wiggled the needle around, trying to start the blood flow, the pain became even worse. The feeling was like an electrical shock, at that moment, I was in an intense amount of pain. I asked her to take the needle out, she said she was almost finished, after wiggling the needle again, the blood finally started going into the vial, she collected it and left the room stating she would be back. I knew then that I had been injured. I completed my visit and left the facility.

I went home still feeling a lot of pain from the blood draw. My hand started to swell, I was hoping it was temporary and would get better soon, it did not, and it became even worse. I felt a tremendous amount of sharp pain, and an electrical shock, after no improvement. I went back to the facility to see the same doctor that I saw there previously; he recommended ice compresses, after going back home again and spending several days doing as the doctor suggested. My injury became even worse. I went to the emergency room at a local hospital, and the doctor there said he believed that I had Venipuncture complex regional pain syndrome II (VPCRPS II), something I had never heard of before. The emergency room doctor recommended I see a Neurologist for further evaluation.

I went back home and researched as much as possible about CRPS, and I went to see a Neurologist. The weeks wore on and the disease started to spread throughout my body. To me it felt like a monster had taken over the inside of my body. The doctor did a nerve conduction test which only aggravated the disease further, and suggested I have a stellate ganglion block (SGB). I learned that it would only treat the initial injured arm. The disease had now spread over a larger area. I decided not to have the treatment and found a Neurologist in Florida. I read about the treatment that he was providing which made sense to me because it would treat my entire upper body. I went to Florida to be evaluated and treated by Doctor HH. He performed a paravertebral epidural nerve block and several trigger point injections, and he prescribed some medications to help treat my disease. Finally, I felt I had some real help, and I felt better than I had since the initial injury and the start of the disease.

I have had the disease for 20-years now, and the pain from it has mostly subsided, but I still have some physical limitations. I believe there is good to be realized with everything. I feel like I have met some wonderful people since being diagnosed. I have met other patients and the medical staff at the doctor's office. Having a diagnosis of CRPS can be so intimidating. The first year or two that I was diagnosed with CRPS, I was scared of what this disease would mean for me. It has now been 20-years since my diagnosis, and I am thankful to maintain it as well as I have.

I often think about patients newly diagnosed with CRPS, and what they are feeling, because I was in their position. It's scary to be diagnosed with a disease for which there is no cure, but dealing with the intensity of the symptoms can be treated. For those of us with CRPS, we can still have long life with it and be given back a better quality of life with the proper treatment. For me that was the most important thing. I felt like the "Monster Within" was able to be controlled.

MY UNBELIEVABLE CRPS STORY:
DESPITE THE PAIN, DEPRESSION, AND LOSS OF MY PRIOR SELF,
I DISCOVERED (THE WHY) THIS HAPPENED AND
HOW I FOUND A WAY TO HELP OTHERS
Cynthia Johnstone Lane

My complex regional pain syndrome (CRPS), also known as reflex sympathetic dystrophy(RSD), began and would change my life in ways I would and could have never thought it would ever turn out to be like this.

My story begins on Thursday February 1, 2001, by checking into our local hospital for what I thought would be a typical in and out hysterectomy surgery. I was one month away from being 33-years-old. I had a husband that I married when I was 17-years-old, we have three children, my daughter Jocelyn 14-years-old, a son Casey nine-years-old, and my youngest son Dalton three-years-old. I had two jobs that I worked so hard to get, and they were my lifelong dreams. I was an LPN(Licensed Practical Nurse) IV certified and was a Sargent in the United States Army Reserve. I was also two weeks away from training to be a medic and get to fly on helicopters. We had also just moved, while I was pregnant, to our new house on an acre of land. We both had wanted this and worked for this so long. We were looking at creating our new life here.

What Started This Life Changing Journey?

Well, I checked in, and did all the pre-surgery things (medical questions asked, consent given, IV started and fluids given) with no incident and talked with my OBGYN Doctor L, before surgery, on what to expect after surgery. All went well with the surgery that I was so ready for. I had for several years of ovarian cysts and monthly pain that would land me in bed for a week or more. My doctor had to go through all the protocols and checklists in order to perform my surgery in our hospital because it was a Nun(Catholic) hospital and insurance wanted numerous tests done before they would pay for it. I remember waking up and my husband and sister-in-law were there in my room. I woke up hurting from incisional pain, needing pain medication which was a little slow coming but my sister-in-law kept the nurses on their toes, until I received it. Shift change came around at 6:00 pm, and my nurse who we will call MJ, came in at some point. I really do not remember her coming in to introduce herself. I was still hooked up to the IV fluids and the IV site was looking good with no issues. I remember waking up around 9:30 pm, and calling for the nurse asking for pain medications. MJ, came in and gave me Demerol/Phenergan, IV pushed fast and cough syrup with codeine. Doctor L, was concerned I could end-up with Pneumonia after some noise was heard in my chest after surgery. At that point, I could feel pain as she was doing the medications through the IV. I said "It burns!" and she said "Oh ya it burns a little " and left. Well that pretty much knocked me out for a few hours till I awoke with MJ, changing the IV fluids about 12:15am. At 12:30 am, I called for pain medications and once again she returned with an IV push of Demerol/Phenergan. This time she did not turn on the bright light to examine the IV site while she pushed the medications. I recall crying out about how bad it burned and she just walked out when she was done. Remember, the IV fluids are on a pump and are being pumped into me all this time. At 3:35 am, the pain from both my incision and my arm woke me up so I rang the nurse again. Once again, she came into my room without turning the light on. I told her of my pain and the pain in my arm.

71

I told her it was cold and it hurt. She still did not turn the light on to look at it. Just a faint little light that I had on all night and the light from the TV is all she used.

She proceeded to push the pain medications through the IV and I cried out to stop, it hurt! It hurt so bad I was crying yet she still did not investigate the site with a better light. Now, to explain a little bit about what would become an issue later on with this IV. Phenergan (anti-nausea medication). At this time, I was given with certain pain medications that were known to cause nausea, so they would give this along with it to help stop some of the nausea and make the pain med more effective as well. Phenergan given through an IV , if infiltrated, can cause tissue damage and or tissue death, depending on the amount given. With that being said and my body absorbing the pain med , I fell back to sleep. "Good Morning " I was woken at about 4:30 am with the next nurse to come on who we will call T. T, came in the room and turned on the bright light and walked over to my bed, where I had a pillow on my belly and my left arm with the IV ,propped up during the night. T, took one look at my arm and said, " OH No!" and proceeded to turn off the pump to the IV. Now my arm was twice the size of the other one and was cold and very painful! I told T, that I had told MJ, that it hurt and she became mad. T, went and had MJ, immediately removed the IV and restarted it in my right wrist. MJ, was not happy about having to restart my IV. She had an attitude and not to mention she was very rude. When Doctor L, came in to see me, he had not learned about what happened yet. He discontinued the IV at that point. He would be releasing me the next day. My arm had already started to looked bruised, and it was still very swollen. By the time I was released it looked like my arm had been in some kind of accident. When I finally, made it home, after a very painful ride, especially for someone who just had their lower insides removed and others moved around, I had to ride in a truck for 15-miles. I do not recommend it! I continued to heal at home, but my arm began to look like and feel like it had been run over. Now, there was more black-and-blue bruising from my wrist up past my elbow, and still double the size. I noticed that I could feel my vein starting to become hard as a rock and very painful. I kept an eye on it the remainder of the week. On, Friday February 9th, I was cold, and was sitting by the fireplace, and I noticed all of my body was mottling(to turn splotchy with bluish coloring) all over. This is something I remembered that people do right before they are going to pass away. My circulation was not right. The pain in my arm was extreme now and the vein was hard from wrist up to elbow, and a red line was now visible. On Saturday February 10th, my Mom and I decided I needed to go to the emergency room (ER) and have it checked out.

So, we did, and I informed the ER what had happened. The ER doctor ordered some labs and an Ultrasound of my arm. I ended up having three doctors come look at it, and at one point they were all arguing about what it could be in front of me. They decided to call an Internal Medicine Doctor in, who I will call Doctor S. He ordered a blood test called a D-Dimer (a test to help rule out the presence of a serious blood clot). It alerts you basically to a blood clot somewhere in your body. Well Doctor S, was also pulled into the augment with the others and he won, and he admitted me due the test was positive, but it was not visible on the ultrasound. Not the first time something wrong was not visible with that test.

So, I waited to go to a room and more people came in to see my arm. I was the talk of the hospital. Lol! Doctor S, had told me he had only treated one other person with a blood clot in their arm, and he had mangled in a car

73

wreck, but that person died because of it. Great, I had a 50/50 chance I could die. I think the odds were greater than that. So, I had yet another IV started in the other arm for Heparin IV to start. Heparin is a blood thinner. This next week the pain I was having was almost unbearable. My arm, I thought they were going to have a cut it off because of the swelling. I thought it was going to burst open. They put some kind of sleeve covering on my arm that would circulate by squeezing off and on to help the swelling go down. During this stay Doctor L, came in and took a look and was not happy that it had happened. After five days of excruciating pain, I was released from the hospital to continue on Coumadin, a blood thinner for the next several months.

As time went on, I healed from surgery and my arm went back to normal size but I could tell and feel something was not right. The pain was still there and now it was burning something fierce. I would return to work after my release was given. My head nurse V, was giving a class on what not to do with an IV's and she took some photos of my arm ,when it happened, to be used for her class. I found out this incident among others was used to stop the use of Phenergan being given through an IV. I would go in weekly for a prothrombin time (PT) test (it is a test that measures how long it takes for a clot to form in a blood sample) at Doctor S, office and I was still taking Lortabs for the pain my arm. I would not take them when I was working. I really tried to work as I had done before surgery, but each day it was getting harder and harder to do.

I had asked several nurses what would happen if I passed part of a clot to my lung known as a Pulmonary Embolism. They told me I could survive but would be lucky and would have to have immediate care if it happened. I do not know why I was asking other than being a nurse. That thought was in the back of my brain, but I never thought of what would happen to me next. I would not know exactly what it was for 10-years.

It was about eight to twelve weeks post-op, and I was back to work now, but was off this morning in question. My husband was getting ready to go to work, and he would leave the house at 5:30 am to be at work at 6:00 am. I made his lunch and just did not feel good. My stomach was nauseated, and I recall my pulse was kind of fast, but I soon became pale and clammy. I went and sat on the side of my bed. I thought I was going to pass out. But I thought of my kids sleeping in the other rooms, and I said I was not going to die here. Then the pain went up my arm and I could not breathe. The pain in my chest was like nothing I had ever felt before. I could not catch my breath. I thought about what could be going on? I yelled for my husband the best I could while trying to catch my breath. He came in, and took one look at me, and knew something was happening that was not good. I had to have help with getting my clothes on and getting into the truck, which was a difficult thing for me to do. He must have driven the fastest he had ever driven to the ER which was 15-20 miles away. The pain was still there but I was able to breathe better by the time we got there. I thought okay, I passed a tiny spec though my lungs. I told the ER about having the blood clot and they ordered a Lung Scan, Blood Test, an Artillery O2 Blood, and a Chest x-ray, but I do not recall having an EKG being done.

I do not like needles whatsoever, so when she went digging for the artery, I came off the table. She tried two times, and she still could not hit the artery. The Doctor said never mind. I was in the ER a few hours and I was sent home. Yes, sent home! I would find out 10-years later after having my yearly physicals, that I had a widow-maker heart attack, and should have been flown to Oklahoma City, to have a heart catheterization done. So, I eventually recover from that visit, and return to work on my next scheduled day, and proceed to put all of this behind us.

Diagnosed

As the months went by, the pain in the arm was just is more than I could handle at times. It was a combination of crushing pain, but I felt a burning pain like it was on fire. My palm would sweat but, the hand was cold. I would mottle and have all kinds of color changes throughout the day. I would return to Doctor S, office monthly, for the prothrombin time (PT) blood test. I would report to him the type of pain I was having, and he was like " I do not know why it is still hurting?" It is healed. But he would still prescribe the Lortabs for me. At night, I would just lay in bed crying holding my arm up in the air because it hurt to touch anything and just the blood pumping through it sent me through the roof. Finally, after months of being in pain, and having no answers as to why Doctor S, would decide to refer me to a neurologist who we will call Doctor V. I went to see Doctor V, and he examined my arm and ordered Neurontin 300 mg daily and physical therapy (PT) three times a week, and gave me a diagnosis of complex regional pain syndrome (CRPS) before I left his office. He also order an EMG, MRI, Bone Scan, and numerous blood tests.

With this diagnosis we returned to Doctor S, office and told him what Doctor V, had said about it being CRPS. Doctor S, had not heard of CRPS so he went and grabbed his PDR(Physician's Desk Reference) and proceeded to look it up. After reading it he slammed the book shut like he did not believe what he had just read. I would go a few more visits to Doctor S, office until he accused me of being a drug seeker, and this pain was all in my head. After I gave him my opinion of him, my husband, and I left and have not been back. This was about June/July of 2001.

Doctor V, did the EMG on my left arm where the IV had been. That was the most painful test I had had done at that point. The little micro-needles injected into my arm were tolerable but when he turned on the machine to do the test, I screamed and started crying. The results showed that my ulnar nerve was dead. This is a nerve that runs on the inner side of your arm on the pinky side. That would make sense since all the fluid and medications shot in my arm while infiltrated pooled on the inside bottom of my arm that night. The MRI, and bone scan showed very little signs of any of the CRPS at that point. But the pain continued to move up my arm at this point. So, Doctor V, decided I needed to go to a pain management doctor to start treatment.

Doctor V, ordered PT three times a week. My favorite thing during therapy was the Aqua pool. I was able to use it when I started PT, and thank goodness my therapist who we will call T, had heard of CRPS, and knew not to do certain things like apply ice at the end of the session. He told me right then at my first visit to remember one thing always, he said "no matter how bad it hurts, keep moving it. He also said what you do not use, you will lose it." What he told me, to this day has stuck in my mind. I would continue with therapy for the next four years. I went as much as I could, to help with movement, and as long as I could tolerate it. I will come back to therapy shortly, to talk about something I hope never happens again.

I made the appointment to see the pain management doctor, and I saw him in June 2001. Then in July 2001, Doctor N, who has his own way of diagnosing CRPS by doing a series of six stellate ganglion blocks(SGB) (A

77

procedure of inserting a needle in the front of your neck, next to your voice box and esophagus to the ganglion nerve bundles on the inside of your spine), and injecting a medication that would block the pain, and basically numb the nerve. He believed that if you had pain relief, no matter how long it was, it was a positive sign for CRPS in his book. I had relief for the first time since this all began. But it would be short lived, only a few hours. I continued doing the other five blocks. I would have one done it every third day. During one of them, I did not get enough medication to keep me asleep, and I woke up when the needle had just reached the nerve bundle. He looked at me and he saw my eyes are open, and said "You are not supposed to be awake!" He said do not move, and give her more medications, and out I went. That freaked me out because I remember it. After all of the blocks, Doctor N, had said "He wished he could have gotten to me sooner." I was given an official diagnosis from Doctor N, in September 2001. Doctor N, had placed me on Elavil, Neurontin, and Thorazine.

Up until now I had been trying to work at my nursing job in a hospital, and was still inactive in the US Army Reserve, due to my pregnancy issues. It had made it difficult to do my weekends, due to the chance I could lose him. I had planned to go back after I healed from the hysterectomy. Over the next three months it got to where I was not able to move patients with my arm hurting. I was working 12-hours a day without pain medications, and it was getting to be too long of a time to handle it anymore. I even tried using a TENS unit while I worked to no avail. My last nursing day was June 19, 2001. That was the day my dreams died. I never thought I would be able to help anyone ever again. That sunk me into what would become a very angry, and depressed person I did not want to be, but it happened.

I continued to see Doctor V, Doctor S, and Doctor N, and now the pain was going up my right arm. Doctor N, said it was time for a spinal cord stimulator(SCS). No, I was not ready or willing to accept that yet. So, my husband J, proceeded to be my researcher and my all-around supporter. He was also my caretaker after procedures. He also drove me all over, to what would become thousands of miles yearly, going to and from doctor's appointments. It took me a long time to look up what CRPS was at that time. My husband would look up different things and bring it home to me to read. We did not have a computer at that time yet. He found an CRPS expert in Texas, that we thought we should try. So, we started our new treatments in March of 2002. It would be a nine-hour drive for us one way, to see them on a monthly basis. We would drive this trip once a month for over a year. We did it, and that is when I was put on a lot of pain medication. Lortab, Zanaflex and Prilosec. My Neurontin had been upped to 900mg, three times a day, Methadone 2.5 up to 5 mg, along with a cancer pain medication that I would swab my mouth with and then had to dispose of it and keep it in a lock box. I was also drug tested monthly to make sure I was taking all the right medications. The pain clinic proceeded to do nerve burning (radiofrequency) and nerve cutting to see if that would help stop the pain signal once they healed and grew back. They would do numerous blocks all over for both upper and lower extremities. At this time my CRPS was in both arms, across my back and chest. I had to have IV' s in my feet when they did a couple of the procedures on both arms and had to stay a week in Texas for all of these medical procedures. They finally concluded, that I needed to have a SCS. So, I searched for a doctor closer to our home for this.

So, in September 2002, I met with Doctor M, to talk about the SCS. I had to go through a trial stimulator. That was very uncomfortable, and painful all in one. But I did have some pain relief. So, we decided that I would get the SCS permanently placed, but first I would have to have a psychological eval to make sure I would not hurt myself with one. So, on October 24, 200, I had my first of two implants. I was very fortunate that Doctor M, was able to place the leads where both my upper, and lower limbs were covered with one machine. The pain at this time went from 10+ down to about a seven, sometimes even lower. Would continue with blocks for breakthrough pain and flare-ups that would happen with the weather change or season changes. Anytime you want to know what the weather was going to do I could tell you pretty much what it would be like. No weatherman needed. Lol!

So, in 2003, I started having upper side abdominal pain after I ate. This went on for months and months. Would go to my local MD, who would order numerous tests, but would it not show or give actual results of what was going on. Finally, I ended up in the ER with severe pain up around the stomach and radiating into the back. So, I was sent to see a surgeon Doctor G. My Gallbladder was in question so, after insurance finally giving the okay, I went in to have it removed. It was Doctor G's, fastest time in a removal of a Gallbladder, under four minutes from start to finish. I stayed in the hospital overnight, and was released the following morning. By now I am not a fan of hospitals or doctors as you can see why. Not even five days after surgery, I was back in the ER with 101-fever. I was so sick! They did some blood tests and was admitted with a staff-infection. I was just beyond upset. I had to stayed in the hospital again for another five days, and I was placed on IV antibiotics. At, this point I was able to educate some of the nurses on CRPS. The pathology report came back on Gallbladder, it was full of cysts, and infection from years of being on the Lortabs, and other medications.

So, to bring you up to speed, I said I would tell you about what happened shortly before I stopped going to PT. I did a total of four years, three times a week. I had woken up one morning and both of my hands were clenched tight in a fist. I could not open them. I immediately called my doctor and PT. Went into the therapist who could not explain how or why they had done this. They worked on both hands and did not get them open! I was just beside myself! It hurt and I just kept having this thought go through my brain that I would not ever use them again! This was not going to happen so I woke up the next morning and proceeded to soak my hands in warm water and tried again to open my fingers. One hand the fingers relaxed just enough I could pop them open. So, I worked on the one hand, and I was able to get the other hand open. I was in severe pain at this point. Then the next morning I did it again. Had to pop them open again. My therapist gave me hand splints to put on in the day time, but it hurt too bad to wear them at night. This went on for two months non-stop every night. Then as fast as it happened, it stopped. The Doctor still does not understand why this happens to me?

My Family and How They Handled My Disease

So, up until now I have not spoken much about my home life, and my children. They suffered through all of this just as much as I did, but I could not see it then. My daughter J, she was 14-years-old when this all took place and she was just into her high school years. I relied a lot on her, and maybe sometimes too much was put on her, and I regret that. She had to watch both of her brothers when I was not able to, which was most of the time. So, she missed so many things that girls her age should be doing, and not having to babysit, clean house, and cook. My mother was also here as well, but would not do certain things, or would let the kids do things, they should have not been doing. To say dysfunctional, we certainly were.

My middle son did not get the attention he should have had during this time, being nine-years-old. So, he would go, and stay at friend's house all the time. He also stayed at my Mothers, who moved into town, about a mile away. Our youngest son who was three-years-old when I got hurt, well somehow, he was the luckiest out of all them. We had given more attention to him than the other two. Not on purpose but he was the baby, and is just laid back, and is an easy-going kid. He does not really remember a lot of what I went through which is a good thing. It was so hard for the older two, and to this day their story and my story are not seen the same way. I just did all I could do with them, with their school activities, and after school activities. I hurt so bad, but they were not always aware of the high amount of pain I was having.

I would say the older two growing up had their moments, and should have been in some kind of therapy, so they could work through their feelings as well , but that is where I failed them. As I look back, I see that would have helped them greatly. Doctor M, asked me one day if I would be interested in helping him with a new support group for families. He thought since my family, and myself had really become educated on this horrid disease, that we all could help other families, and just maybe my kids could receive some type of support too. So, the kids, my husband, and myself drove 150 miles one way, sometimes monthly, to speak to other families who had a loved one with CRPS. I have learned through all of this that talking to others who are going through the exact same issues, does a world of good for both parties. Talking things out is the best therapy I think there is.

To express, and let your feelings be known to each other opens up the lines of communication to let everyone know how you are feeling, and how they are feeling too. It also helps to educate others in the family who may not be complete believers of this disease. Many spouses of the CRPS suffer have a hard time processing that your wife or husband cannot do certain things anymore, or are not the same person anymore. So, they become depressed as well. My husband has been to every one of my doctor's appointments, and procedure I have had done. The other partner needs to be there to learn, and discuss with the medical team what is going on, and what they will be doing to the one with CRPS.

I have learned to not ever go to a doctor visit or hospital visit without having someone with me. It is much safer to always have another set of eyes and ears there when you cannot be alert. My husband, I have to thank him for all he has done for me in supporting me through this. He has seen me at my worst and at my best, and he still to this day, still goes with me. No, it has not always been easy, and we had our moments. A sickness will stress the very core of any family. That is where the communication comes in.

I do believe we were able to help some other families in understanding what we, who have CRPS, go through daily. Not sure if the group is still together, but I hope so. I sometimes wish I could go back in time, just like everyone does. I would, if I could. I would have tried to see my kid's point of view, and what they were feeling.

I was in too much pain, and most of the time they would see me in bed sleeping, or on so many pain medications that I was not able to do anything. That brings me to something a doctor said to my husband when I was going to Texas monthly for treatments and appointments. The doctor had mentioned all the medications I would be on, and my husband asked "Doc, well what about her becoming addicted to the pain medications?" The doctor proceeded to tell J , " That was the least of his worries, he was just trying to keep me alive." He said that I was going to become physically addicted, and that just happens after you have been on this amount of medication for a certain amount of time. The difference is mentally we are not addicts. The doctor was worried that I may try to at some point, if he did not keep my pain down, try to end it all.

This disease is also known as the Suicide Disease because of the pain we are in daily. I cannot say, that thought did not cross my mind, because I did hurt beyond anyone's comprehension. But my husband, and kids are what kept me moving forward to try to hold on the best I could.

Now Doctor M, did an awesome job with my stimulator and I could not, at this time, charge the battery up on this model. So, when the opportunity came around, and my power level was getting low, Doctor M, thought I should upgrade my SCS to a newer improved device that I could charge the battery myself. By using an attachment that would lay across the battery which was in my right buttock. It would take about an hour, depending on how low the battery was. So, I did the surgery, and placement was as good as the first time. I really liked the new SCS, and was able to get a little bit better relief. Had no issues with the incisions, at least I did not think so? I had the SCS for about a year ,and the area around the battery started to hurt and was getting warm.

Well, I started to notice that I had some oozing occasionally on my underwear that should not be there. So, I put some antibiotic cream on it, and it stopped shortly after. Well then about a week later the area was swollen and puffy, so I pushed on it. Nasty yellow gunk came out a tiny hole, and by the next day I had a red streak starting up my back and I was running a 101 fever. I immediately called Doctor M, and he had to do an emergency removal due to an infection going up my back. He had to get it stopped, and out before it went to the spinal cord area. He ordered antibiotics, and said I must have had a pin hole in the incision where the battery was that never healed. I think it was a staple that was missed. So, every time I took a bath, water would get in it and start the infection.

Doctor M, had mentioned he noticed something strange on my cardiac monitor during surgery, but since it was there every time he did a procedure, he really did not think much of it. I never had any issues during any procedures when it came to my heart. So, he just left it alone.

So, after the stimulator came out, Doctor M, wanted to veer away from prescribing the pain medications for routine prescribing so he referred me to a pain management/psychologist Doctor B. This would be different as I would go in, and sit in his office, and he would ask how my pain was. He would ask if I was having any other issues, and then write my prescriptions. Would never do any vitals, or any kind of physical exam. He would send me yearly to get a physical at my GP's office, and receive the results.

No one ever heard, or if they did, they never followed through on what was heard in my chest. They never asked me anything either. So, at this point in May of 2005, I was on Neurontin 800mg four times a day, Cymbalta 60mg daily, Ambien 10mg nightly, Tizanidine 4mg three times a day,

Oxycodone 10 three times a day, Fentanyl 75mcg patch every three days, Temazepam 30mg twice a day, and Morphine 15mg. I was on all of this, and still my pain was a 10+. I would continue seeing Doctor B, for the next five years. I did what I could do.

Being on all of these medications I gained 50+ pounds. Of which did not help my pain. I was still able to drive somewhat around locally, but anything long distance was difficult, and I tried not to do it, but I also tried to live my life, and give my kids some kind of life that did not involve seeing mom in bed all the time. I would periodically have nerve blocks done by Doctor M, when a flare-up would not calm down. Doctor M, was really wanting me to consider having a morphine pump implanted but I was not doing that yet. I was still too young to even consider that yet. So, I said to him no, not yet.

When I stopped working in June 2001, I immediately filed for Social Security Disability Insurance (SSDI). I filed, and was denied the first time. Then I hired a law firm to help me appeal the decision. No one knew what CRPS was at that time, but finally, they received a diagnosis coding number depending on whether you had Type I or Type II CRPS. That would help so many people finally get approved for their benefits. It was hard trying to make ends meet since we lost one paycheck, and the chance for another one was also gone. So, the kids, and us would have to go without things to get by.

We did not go out to eat, go to the movies, or take vacations. So, the kids did not get to experience many family trips. I would be denied two more times for my disability. I could not believe that they thought I could work, and do it safely on all of the medications I was on, let alone be able to physically handle it. That would be a Big No, and so finally after a long drawn out battle a judge finally approved me for it in September 2005. That was a Godsend when that happened. My husband' s insurance had been covering everything medical wise, but it would be nice to have the extra insurance as well. So, my children also received a portion of my benefits as well monthly.

Life at this point consisted of me getting up to make my husband's lunch, and wake the kids for school. I would then lay back down, and would get up around 9:00 am or so, and would take all my medications for the morning. It was very difficult just with regular movement, and just taking a shower daily, was an ordeal. I would have to lay down from just doing that. This is no way to live. The pain was so unbearable all I could do was just lay there because any movement, stress, or exertion just compounded my pain, and added even more to the depression that now was my life, or what I had left of my life. I did not like who I had become, or what my life was like so each day I would sink deeper into a darker place. When you' re in pain either physically, or mentally all you want is it to stop. I wanted my old life back! Why did this happen to me! I worked so hard to get where I was, and I just went in for a routine surgery, and in one night, my whole life was turned upside down, and sideways. I am still upset to this day. I had so many plans that were just destroyed that night. Still hard to believe, but I know there had to be a reason, but I would pray nightly asking God what was the reason, and why? I would find out what, I think the "why" was in a few more years down the road.

Looks Can Be Deceiving

To look at me from the outside you would think there was not anything wrong with me other than I moved, and walked slowly because my feet hurt. I did have to go to a podiatrist because my toenails were growing in towards themselves like an inverted V. It was very painful, and I could not wear shoes for very long, or at all. So, I went in and had surgery done on both feet. I decided to have both done at the same time to deal with the pain all at once, instead of dragging it on. They removed every toenail on one foot and three on the other foot. Oh my God it hurt like hell! I had to be careful, and keep it clean, and when the nails grew back-in, they were so much better. But when you have CRPS one thing is our nails can grow thicker, and thicker, and so that happened to me again.

From the time of being diagnosed, or shortly after when I was able to look up this disease, and not get emotional, I looked for support groups to talk with others who had what I had, and that did help me knowing they knew what I was feeling and that we were all in the same boat. I was able to find a local in-person group, that I attend monthly but started to dwindle down as people just stopped participating in it.

So, I eventually found one on the computer in the city I would go to see my doctor. It was online but some would meet in person at times. I was in that group for about a half a year, then one of the main administrators could not handle the pain, and overdosed. That was my first time dealing with that type of grief. I stopped participating in the group shortly after. I understand why people do it but, what they do not get is the chain of events they create when they do it. The family members, and children, if they have any, are left with a lifetime of pain, and wanting to understand why they did it. It also can set up other members to be so depressed, and sad that they may do the same thing. Thinking they cannot handle their pain either. But there are times when people have accidently overdosed (OD), or had other health issues, and that is very hard to take as well. I have lost a few friends I have met online that had CRPS, or a chronic pain disorder that are no longer here. I make sure they all know I care and will always be here for them. We are not alone, and no one should ever feel that they are alone, or think no one understands what they are going through.

To briefly touch on how I handled what little bit, we did travel. We went to the Gulf Coast for a family week with my dad, brother, and sister. Along with their families and stayed in a beach house for a week. Well, it took us about 12-hours to get there and that was stopping overnight because of all of the little ones we all had. By the time we arrived I was in so much pain that I was physically sick for two of those days. I mean nausea and vomiting sickness with pain. I have never been like that before. Even my husband did not understand how I was so sick. My family actual saw for the first time how bad I was at that point. Not sure if they ever truly believed that I had something wrong with me or not. We would go on a few other trips. Had to fly to Pennsylvania to be evaluated by an CRPS expert, and I had to stay overnight because of what traveling did to me. It was not as bad as the driving, but it would still send me into a flare-up.

Meeting Our Life Saver

Had been watching the news one night in 2010, and heard about a doc who they were looking for because some of his patients had been caught selling their pain medications . Well, come to find out it was my pain management Doctor B. I was like OMG! What am I going to do now? So, I called Doctor M, and he said he would refer me to someone else. So, I set up an appointment with my new pain management doctor who we will call

Doctor P. We went to my first appointment and I met him. He was very pleasant, with an easy-going bedside manner, and a jokester as well (of which grows on you through the years. Lol!) He also would inform me how he would take off several weeks in the summer because he traveled with Doctors Without Borders. Which just put another check mark in the approval box for him.

Finally, one I did not have to either educate or put up with them thinking they knew more about than myself. He stood there and let me tell him all I had been through. Then he says to me I am going to make you feel better! I looked at my husband and we both laughed. Yes, we heard that before! I did not believe him but was willing to give it a try for a short time.

He proceeded to do my labs and did a DEXA Scan(Bone Density Scan) to check the bone thickness and to monitor any bone loss from here on out. I stayed on all of the same medications I was on and he added one but it did nothing for me that first month. He checked my hormones and started me on hormone replacement as well. He listened to my heart and said he heard something like a strange murmur and thought I should have an ultrasound done asap. Was scheduled and we returned to have it done. Then followed up the next month when he asked me when I had my heart attack? I looked at him like," What did you say?" He asked when did I have a heart attack? I said, "It had to have been in 2001." Also stated it had been a widow-maker and I was very lucky to have still been here. He was going to send me to one of the best Cardiologists in the state, Doctor H. At, this point my jaw is on the floor! A heart attack? Really, I was just 42-years-old at this point so I was 33-years-old when I had it and was never told by the hospital it had happened.

So, during my second visit, as though finding out about the heart attack was not enough, Doctor P, had started me on one medication and wanted me to try it for the CRPS and it did nothing for the pain of the CRPS. So, Doctor P, told us about an article he had just read about using this medication that would increase the dopamine levels and had been known to decrease the CRPS pain in studies. Said it was a Parkinson's medication called Mirapex (Pramipexole) but I would have to go up slowly on it.

So, I agreed to try it. At this point I had nothing to lose. He also wanted me to stop smoking. I was up to a pack and a half a day. Smoked since I was 15. Boy, this would be difficult with the pain I was in and now the stress of knowing what the smoking was doing to me and my heart. I was determined to quit so I started out trying the Chantix. Well first month okay, but second month I had to stop. Was having strange thoughts and I did not like that.

So, I returned after the first month being on Mirapex. Something was changing but I wasn't sure and did not want to hope too much. I also started on Wellbutrin and Nicotine patches to try again with the smoking issue. Would take a total of three times of trying to quit too finally do it! I was a non-smoker! Yes!

So, the following month there were big changes with my pain levels with the Mirapex. I went from .125mg up to 3mg in two months. Really had no issues going up slowly, but after hitting the 3mg I was walking around the house doing stuff, like cleaning and my activity had increased and I stopped for a minute and yelled at my husband. I couldn't be sure and did not want to jinx myself and was thinking this was a short-lived response but I was PAIN FREE for the first time in 10-years! I just started crying and so did my husband! I called and made an appointment to see Doctor P, to tell him. I

91

had noticed though as I was going up the last part of the Mirapex to the 3mg, that I was decreasing the pain medication I was on. Just did not need them, so I took less daily. I eventually weaned myself off them when my pain was gone and quit smoking to boot.

So, Doctor P, had scored an A+ and became my life saver and life giver all with this medication! I was in shock and he was too, I think. We all were crying together! So along with the pain being gone the symptoms of the CRPS started to go away. No more mottling, no more skin changes and my toenails went back to normal. My life was given back to me for the most part, I thought. But I would find out about six months later that it is not in remission , it was still very active in my body. It is just being controlled so to speak with the medication. I had run out and was having issues with a nurse to reorder it. Took about three weeks to get back on it, but after the first four to five days, I was right back to a 10+ pain level and no pain medication to speak of. I said never again will this happen. I started back and the pain was gone again. Thank you, God! This happened in 2011.

So, while I was going up on the Mirapex, our air conditioner broke down that summer and we were three to four days without the cool air in 100+ degree days. One of our hottest summers. Well, I did not think much of it and there was not anything I really could do. I hurt too much to do anything so I lay down in bed with a fan on me, and thought I was fine. We fixed the air as soon as we could, and went on about our life. The kids started noticing I would fall off the bed when I was just sitting there. They thought, "Oh Mom is taking too much pain medications." No, I was not though. I was standing in the kitchen one night getting something out of the top cabinet and last thing I knew I was on the floor. I just went out, and did not know why? I called Doctor P, the next day, and went there for a visit. He did some labs, and we came home. I got a call the next day from Doctor P, asking me how long it would take me to get back down to the city? I asked him why what was wrong? He said my kidneys had quit working, and were trying to restart but they could not. He was going to admit me into the hospital, and he had called a Kidney specialist.

Along with my pain decreasing I had my first visit with Doctor H, the cardiologist who wanted me to have a heart catheterization done to see what kind of damage was done to my heart. Had it done they went through my groin to do this one and he had also ordered an ultrasound to measure the amount my heart was pumping out to my body. My ejection rate or Cardiac Output.

Most people pump out at 50%-70% being healthy. Most heart patients are somewhere around 30-25% giving their diagnosis. Mine was at 10-15% Output. Was not on O2, but would end up on it for a short time at night. The results of heart catheterization showed that the bottom of my heart did not work! It is basically dead and doesn't pump! The doctor was amazed that I was actually not showing a lot of signs of it. I had lived with it so long that I was used to it but he knew that would change soon. I was at extreme high risk for a second heart attack that I would not survive. The Doctor said I needed a pacemaker defibrillator soon. One of the main blood vessels on the heart muscle itself had been blocked and could not be stunted now. The damage was done. I was thrown back and scared to death! I said how and what I could do to not need one? They said to get my ejection percentage (Cardiac Output) up to 32% or higher. So, I set out to do it.

Picking back up with the kidneys, which pretty much happened at the same time. The Doctor was not sure why my kidneys just quit only that they could not restart on their own so, I started on bicarbonate-based medications of which I had my first ever picc line! I had helped with those and did not want to get it. But after years of having CRPS my veins had just gone to crap with all the treatments, and procedures I had done. I recovered and returned home after a week in the hospital and proceeded to drop my weight and increase my cardiac output. I did not want the pacemaker. So, the next year I was able to drop 50-pounds and increase my cardiac output up to 31%. I could not hit the 32%, I wanted to not have to have one. I was devastated and scared beyond anything anyone could imagine. I gave in, and scheduled the pacemaker to be implanted. Little did I know just how badly the defibrillator would come into being used.

So, you know how stress is a killer, well this day it would prove itself. I was driving into town about a mile from my house to pay a city bill. I get to my first turn and do not feel real, good, but I slow down to make the turn. Then all of a sudden, I feel what I describe as an explosion in my chest and immediate pain. I thought and said "Oh God just help me get some help and do not let me die right here!" I make it there and proceed to get out of my car and go inside. I walked up to the desk and said I think I need an ambulance! They sat me down and lucky enough an EMT was close by and came to do my vitals. My blood pressure (B/P) was some ungodly amount like 240/180. I was scared and had them call my friend to come get my car and to call my husband please. I really thought I was dying. More EMT's come in while waiting for the ambulance. This would be my first time in one. Lol! They loaded me up and started an IV, and luckily, I had a paramedic with us who could give the morphine for pain and was given several doses of nitro.

I got to the hospital. and immediately is admitted into the ICU where we wait till my pacemaker can be downloaded. The tech had to come from the southern part of the state which was like 250-miles away. Only one at that time for the whole state. He gets there, and downloads it. Well, this is why they wanted me to have one. They knew it was just a matter of time and I would have a major heart attack again.

They read out the memory on the pacemaker, and said my heart was just fluttering between 600-800 beats per minute, and so I was shocked back into rhythm. I was shocked with the full-amount of joules! That is the amount of shock you receive. That was 360 joules and approximately 16-amps. The machine had not been regulated yet. It was less than a year after getting it that it shocked me. So, it bruised the inside of my chest wall and I was in pain for about half a year from it. I had it regulated after that but later on in 2012, I would once again be shocked and spend the night in ICU close to Christmas time.

How I Still Can Help Others

When they say you have guardian angels around, believe it. One of them just happens to have MD/GP behind his name. I call him my life saver literally! I would not be here if it had not been for Doctor P. He heard something that no other doctors for 10-years heard of was concerned about. I continue to not be in CRPS pain, and I want to tell others about (this gift from God is what I call it) this medication, so I start talking about it in a support group on Facebook. People with CRPS learn to be, by no fault of their own, very skeptical of others who say they do not have pain, because of a treatment or medication. We just do not believe it anymore. We become so tired and have been let down so many times that it is hard to believe anyone. Not to mention the amounts of medications tried on us to no avail. So, when I start talking about this medication, I get a message from the administrator of the group that I would have to stop talking about the medication I was on. That I was advertising it. I said if I cannot talk about it how would anyone know? Was told they could go back in history on the page and find it. I asked, ``How will they know it is there if I cannot tell them about it for them to look up?" I said what kind of support group stops someone from possibly helping someone else? I do not think they believed me about it or my story.

So, I continued to ask questions and they both got mad and threw me out. I was just devastated that I was thrown out of a support group trying to help others. It made no sense to me at all. So, that depressed me. I just stopped using Facebook at that point. Then one day I thought to myself about three months later, why do not I start my own group?

So, in 2014, I started a group called CRPS/CRPS Warriors-Help & Support For Your Daily Battles. I have 604 members and growing as of 2021.

My Thoughts About Getting CRPS

So, to say my life changed in ways I could have never thought back then when I was diagnosed with CRPS, that I could not have been even close to thinking about it like this. This is why we have to keep believing that one day a cure or even just a medication like I am on will help all of us with CRPS.

No matter how bad you feel, you cannot give up. I believe God uses us and has our life planned out. I had to go through all I did in order to help others. Until, you have lived with CRPS, others who do not have it do not understand. When you tell them about CRPS, it usually go in one ear and out the other. They have no clue about this type of pain and depression we live with. So, I had to understand CRPS in order to help others. I lived it and know the pain and know the looks that I receive from people because they do not believe you are sick. So, God has a plan and we do not always find out what that plan is, so I could be wrong but, he has kept me here on earth for some reason. I believe it is to pass on to and help others as I have. I will continue to educate others on a medication that may be their life changer, and along with all the treatments and procedures available. Also, along with what to look for as in adverse results that can happen.

MY CRPS JOURNEY
Karey Stanziale

My complex regional pain syndrome (CRPS) journey started when I was only 19-years-old. This is when my life changed in an instant. I went in for surgery to repair a herniated disc at L-3/L-4 level, and going into that surgery I was otherwise a healthy woman.

On January 9, 2000, my life would change forever. Now, I am a 22-year full body and internal organ CRPS warrior. I was just a kid when a Neurosurgeon from Yale New Haven Hospital damaged my sciatic nerve during surgery to repair a herniated disc.

I remember being a nervous wreck before the surgery, but I knew that my family was there waiting for news on how my surgery would go.

I do not remember how long the actual surgery went, but I remember waking up seeing my surgeon standing over me. He smiled and said that everything had gone well and he would see me in a few weeks as he was off for vacation. He told me his nurse would take care of anything I needed. I remember my head clearing enough to inquire about my right leg-my feeling in it was GONE. He told me not to worry that I had had numbness before with my previous surgery and everything would be okay. Well, it was not okay. My life changed forever in that instant.

The early onset of pain was tough. I could not stand, and I could not walk. Every time I tried my leg gave out completely. I could not even hold my own weight. I was scared to death over the whole situation.

Three weeks later I was in the doctor's office getting the staples he used for my incision out. My leg was still completely numb and my right foot was drooping I could not move it normally anymore. He did his examination, and told me I had developed foot drop on the right side, and would have to be fitted for a leg brace, so I did not trip over it while trying to walk.

This was the onset of my CRPS. My life has never ever been the same since. That constant burning pain started from that surgery, which went from my back down my right leg and into my toes. My surgeon did a bunch of tests, and told me that my sciatic nerve was damaged during surgery, and that once it healed by itself, I would be okay. Well, it never healed. It took me 17-long-years before I was properly diagnosed with CRPS by a doctor.

Before my diagnosis the doctor blamed my pain on everything else, even though I was screaming about my symptoms from the onset, immediately after my surgery.

They've claimed it was just depression, or that I had become addicted to pain killers. One doctor told my family I was addicted to opioids, and that I would never get better. I was told that a lot over the years that I was making things up, and that it was all in my head. How I hated hearing that after a while.

I played the pass around game from doctor to doctor for 13-years after my surgery. When the surgery first happened, I had private insurance, and it covered things like physical therapy and chiropractic appointments which also included doing a deep tissue massage every time I went. The treatments truly helped me, and I got on with my life. The pain was not gone, and I immediately had a temperature-differences in both legs.

I remember borrowing a friend's nail polish one day that was a different color depending on the temperature of your nails. I remember doing my toes, and my right toes were purple my left a bright neon pink. It was because my right leg from the day of that surgery felt dead. It felt cold as a corpse, it has been that way for almost 23-years now. It is funny how some people would ask me why on earth would I paint my toes different colors? They did not believe when I said the polish was heat sensitive, and it just came out that way when I polished them due to my cold foot and leg.

One day everything changed for me. It was right before Christmas 2013, and I got a phone call from a random radiologist who asked me if I had any incontinence issues? I told him that I had been having issues with my bladder, but I could not get a neurologist to look at me, and my urologist had done everything he could think of besides remove my bladder to fix whatever the problem was. He even agreed it was not my bladder.

The radiologist said I had to call a Neuro-oncologist at Yale and that he could provide the answer, and the reason for my incontinence. He was kind to give me the doctor's name and phone number, so I did call this doctor. Three days later I walked into the Neuro-oncologist office, and he tells me that I have cauda equina syndrome, and that the roots of the tumor were strangling the nerves to my bladder causing the urine incontinence. I had been experiencing this for years at that point.

What was more disturbing is that he could see the tumor as far as 13-years before, on some old MRI films. He could not believe that none of my neurologists or surgeons had seen it. He referred me to the surgeon who would be assisting in the surgery to get it off of my spine. At this point I was absolutely terrified.

I met the team of nurses and doctors who would be on the "A" team for my care. I immediately got asked why I waited so long to have the tumor removed. They were shocked to learn that I had absolutely no idea the tumor was even there. I am not the kind of person to ever neglect anything medically. I learned a long time ago with this monster, and even before I was diagnosed to not have it checked out. Sometimes it is nothing, however in my experience most of the time something is wrong, and I am glad I went to see this doctor.

Anyhow they had me go for a full body MRI of my spine to make sure the only tumor I had was the one they found.

Let's fast forward six months. After having my full body MRI, I went for my follow-up exam with the doctor and he told me that MRI had showed the tumor had grown 2cm, and it absolutely had to come out because it was strangling the nerves to my bladder leaving me completely urine incontinent. This was the cause of my problem. Because it had grown so much in so short amount of time, it had to come out.

July 9 2014, was my fourth surgery to remove the tumor from my spinal cord. Going in I was terrified. Coming out I was so much better the urine incontinence stopped immediately, and I was so happy the surgery had help me.

Two weeks later I was in the emergency department again. I had a spinal fluid leak and meningitis. Now, I had to have surgery number five.

After recouping from those surgeries, I went to see my Neuro-oncologist who told me that they removed the cancer, and that I would not need any further treatments, because they got the root as well. I have been cancer free for seven years. Thank God!

It was around this time that I was finally diagnosed properly with CRPS. My oncologist is the one who properly diagnosed me. He is a very prominent Neuro-oncologist at Smilow Cancer Hospital in New Haven, CT.

The Creation of a Star Named Courage

Dealing with what happened to me, I was so angry. I went through absolute hell trying to get diagnosed for over 15-years. The diagnosis floored me, and I felt so alone.

So, my search began on Facebook to find others like me in the hopes of finding help. What I found was the most loving, and supportive group of people I have ever met. Eager to share their stories, and experiences. They gave me the hope to fight back, and fight to obtain better doctors.

This is where everything changed for me. It is where I found my tribe on Facebook, and the WONDERFUL supportive CRPS family there have saved my life more times then, I ever care to admit.
I swore that I would find a positive way to unite all 2.5 million of us in a positive way, so we would know without a doubt that we were not alone in this world. That's one of the things I saw being posted about on many CRPS groups on Facebook.

Last march Covid-19 exploded worldwide, and all of us felt the uncertainty far worse, because not only were we feeling isolation, and uncertainty of being diagnosed with CRPS, we suddenly found our worlds become so much smaller in a world of face masks and self-isolation. Covid-19 was and is still the worst illness to ever hit humanity.

So, one night I was watching the Mandy Moore movie called: A Walk to Remember. In the movie there is a character who buys a star for his girlfriend, who is terminally ill with cancer. It suddenly it crossed my mind. How perfect would that be if we had a star, something so positive it would bring hope to all of us, and it would be a way to leave my legacy for both of my children. Not only would I be the warrior they watch get up over and over again, no matter how many times my CRPS knocked me down. I was the woman in their life that would always get back up no matter what the situation was. They have been my reason to stand, and fight against this awful disease. I wanted to give not only to them, but to all of the CRPS warriors worldwide. I wanted to give something that would be so positive it would make a difference for all of us. So, I placed us in the stars. Courage is her name and she is for all of us worldwide, because nobody knows what courage really is until you get diagnosed with this beast, we call CRPS. Now none of us are alone, and it is also for my kids too. Heaven forbid I get called to heaven; they will never be alone. So, now we all can just look up into the sky to see the star named Courage.

I would like to give a huge thank you to Eric Phillips, for letting me submit my story. It truly means they world to me, and I hope it can be an inspiration for just one person to not give up.

APRIL'S CRPS JOURNEY
April Ball

My name is April Ball, and I was originally injured after riding a mountain coaster in Gatlinburg, TN in July of 2016, and then ended up with a herniated disc at L5/S1. After going through all the physical therapy, and seeing a chiropractor, with none of that working for me, and the doctors saying that surgery was not an option because the herniation was not enough to deem surgery, they wanted to try epidural injections, so we went that route. The first injection worked great, and I felt wonderful for about six weeks. After that I had to go back for another injection. That second injection did not help at all, so about four weeks later, my pain management doctor was setting me up for another epidural injection. Before getting this third injection done, he talked to me about how he was going to do it different than the other two. In his words, he was going to get straight to the source. He was going to go right at the disc this time to help with the pain. This was around February 2017. My husband took the day off, and was sitting right outside of the room I was in getting the injection done. Once I was settled, and the doctor started, I was fine, and then the next thing I know I was screaming in pain, and it felt like I was being stabbed with a knife in the small of my back, and then it was being ripped down my right leg. My husband said he could hear my scream. The doctor had to give me extra pain medication in order for me to go home.

Twenty-four hours later, I was unable to turn my head, change my clothes, or get myself to the bathroom without assistance. My husband called the office where I had the injection, and the doctor on call had us go to the emergency room (ER) immediately. He felt maybe I had a reaction to the injection, or possibly needed to be checked for meningitis. He called ahead for us, and we got in immediately. I was given a spinal tap, which was clear for meningitis. But I was still having issues of not being able to walk, my head hurt, my right leg was burning like hell, and it was red. I felt like I was in overall hell for the couple of days in the hospital. I was kept for observation. After that it was like my life went downhill with no answers. That third epidural was the onset of my complex regional pain syndrome (CRPS), but at that time we did not know that. It took almost a year for me to get diagnosed with CRPS by the same doctor that gave me the epidural injection.

I have had CRPS since February 2017, and I had tried so many medications that have not worked. I have also had a spinal cord stimulator (SCS) implanted in March of 2019, in hopes that would help me with my pain level. It only made things worse, and made my CRPS spread. So, the SCS was removed in April 2021. So, it is pretty easy to say that it was the third epidural injection I had caused the onset of my CRPS. This disease has also spread into my internal organs, such as my stomach, my intestines, and my pancreas. It has caused my pancreas to stop working and producing enzymes. I was on medication for that, but then that stopped working for me also. My pancreas always feels like a punching bag. Having full body CRPS is not fun at all!

Once I was diagnosed with CRPS, I was started on medications for nerve pain, and I also had a couple of nerve blocks, and with the SCS implanted in March 2019, which only made my CRPS worse, and made it spread, we knew it was not going to work, and only made my pain even worse. Another reason for the removal is I was also being tested for multiple sclerosis (MS). Good news with that is, I do not that have it on top of this monster.

I have not taken any type of opioid for my pain. I do love my CBD. I also have an amazing service dog that helps me with my balance and mobility, being that I have falls and stumble a lot.

I was working when I was diagnosed with CRPS. I lost a good job because the owner said I was a liability to the company with my limp. He said to me that he did not want me to sue him if I fell. I was like, REALLY MAN!!! You have to be kidding me? But I have stayed positive throughout my CRPS journey. I have had my ups and downs with it. I have my meltdowns because I am slowly losing my independence. I have an amazing husband who is my rock. I could not ask for a better man to walk with me through this. He is always had my back through everything. This has been the worst thing I have ever been through and I could not do it without him.

Having this disease is tough on the warrior, when their family does not understand what you are going through. When you are in this agony of pain and they treat you like it is all in your head. They get mad when you cannot attend family gatherings sometimes because you are in so much pain you are sick you your stomach. I have family that tries to compare their pain to mine. What do you do? What do you say? They are not understanding how bad my quality of life as gone down. I have begged my doctor to take my bad leg, so that I can have a better quality of life. All my family can say is do not do it, you will regret it, that will be a big mistake. They keep asking me if I still want my leg off. Well yeah! I do have some family members that have learned about CRPS, to be able to help me through my journey. But I also have family that refuse to learn about this disease but either listening to me or by researching it. Once I was learning to understand it more and to bring more awareness about CRPS, in the month of November, when it's CRPS Awareness month. I was told by a family member that I was letting my CRPS consume my life, and that I needed to start my own page about CRPS, and only invite people who really cared because no one really cares about me having CRPS. I have never had any words hurt me has much as those did in my life. Especially coming from the one who said it. That was in the beginning and now we do not have a relationship. It breaks my heart so bad.

Over these past few years, I have been doing what I can to get my non-profit going, and I have been making my goodies for CRPS Warriors, and helping make a difference. Since having Leo, my service and starting Leo's CRPS Awareness and Goodies, it has also helped me. I feel I have a purpose, and that purpose is advocating, and bringing awareness to CRPS!

April Ball

#CRPSWarrior

BEAUTY AND THE BEAST AND HOW I KEEP IT CONTAINED!
Elisabeth Warner

My name is Elisabeth Warner and I'm writing this story to tell you about my experience with having complex regional pain syndrome (CRPS).

My story first started in the late 1990s, when I fell on my head in a boat mishap while working as a fisheries biologist for the Maryland Department of Natural Resources. That was the beginning of the end of everything for what I will refer to as the old me. My career, my marriage, my dreams, and being the best mom ever was all hanging in the balance the day. I ruptured a disc and eventually needed surgery in 2000, or maybe I did not? I got talked into it by the orthopedist, I will never know, I would choose a different path if I had to do it over. I ended up needing a second surgery to replace another disc after, I herniated the discs above and below the original fusion. No one cared to change my job duties in human resources, and I think my doctor did not understand my level of physicality of the job. In 2003, they put new screws, and cadaver bone in, and when I woke up from that, I felt a dull aching pain in my right arm that was new to me, and now I never thought it could be with me for the rest of my life. I tried my hardest living with myself and my arm after that surgery. I tried to go back to work but my job was to drive around the state towing boats and people all over the Chesapeake Bay to surveys at all hours. This was my dream job, I told my parents when I was a pre-teen, I wanted to work for DNR and save the fishes, and here I was.

When I originally injured myself, it was a work-related injury, so I had to use Worker's Compensation(WC) for my treatment and battled them for every bit my care. You would think they were there for you as an employee, but they were not. They were there for the State of Maryland. Injured Workers Insurance Fund (IWIF) was the insurance company. It's a big corporation, so they had no idea what was going on with my case at any time. If it wasn't for my supervisors and friends on the job, I could have lost my job and my mind, luckily my supervisors were probably the best people in my life. They supported me through everything, and if I couldn't get to work on time I could come and stay late, or I could work at home and they were able to allow me to be a good worker still. I always had good reviews, as the one thing that I always appreciated and couldn't live without was my job. My co-workers and my supervisors were my family. At, this point it was me, myself, and I. My family only cared I was on pain medications, and muscle relaxers, and all the rest of the medications they try. They thought I was just home eating Bonbons, wasted on pills, and not working.

I was out for my second surgery, I was trying to heal and ready to get back to work, mentally , I was always one to jump back into work right away. When it was time to return, I did, I found some office work on the computer that I could work on indoors. I started having trouble right away with my neck and shoulders cramping and burning. I could barely last 10-minutes without having to stop and lie down and rest my neck. Pain meds were hardly affecting my pain. I kept trying to work, my doctor put me on half days, which was one of the hardest struggles in my life because my job was my identity. Why can't I get better? I had stayed home and I did everything I was supposed to, the therapy and stretches and kept feeling a weird pain in my right arm, the more I moved the angrier the pain and it became like a toothache, not much would make it go away. By this point, sleep was not an option and this monster we call CRPS was ruining everything and was really interfering with every aspect in my life. At, the time of my second surgery, I was going through some other severe mental

109

stresses including being stalked by my (now) husbands, sister, and his teenage children who wanted me gone. That was the start of my PTSD. I still to this day puke when I see or hear about them. I wonder what effect these stresses had on my healing process, whether the combination of the emotional stress plus the surgery had something to do with the outcome of this crazy complex regional pain syndrome. I may never know.

Once my surgeon realized the fusion failed, he abandoned me and sent me to pain management, there was no explanation for my crazy pain and there was nothing he could do, but write a note that I can't work in this condition, and no one knew what to do next. After they had me on pain medicines that were not doing anything, I knew something was really wrong. My arm throbbed at will multiple, times an hour, day and night and was unbearable I went back to the doctors. they upped my pain meds, and just didn't take it seriously and didn't understand how much it was affecting my life.

At this point, it was getting to where I had to go back to my job because you have to go back at some point if WC insists, unless you have a good lawyer, which I found out later I was a much better advocate for myself, than my lawyer was. I still plan on writing the bar a letter in complaint.

Luckily, my IWIF commissioner heard me, and attempted to advocate for me expertly. I refused to listen when my lawyer said to just go back to work and try, and the commissioner took my side.

My supervisors were awesome throughout this time, exactly the opposite of the insurance company. They gave me alternate duties to try if I could. My right arm which I type with was barely unusable and I couldn't even sit in chair for 20-minutes. I tried to work with voice activated software but it was not like the modern software that's easy and fast. Thru this process, I am on like major painkillers, embarrassingly huge amounts of painkillers which I did not take them all, or I surely would not be here today. The job of WC doctors, is to get you back to work, they did not care that I would be driving eight other people or less or more at 2:00 a.m., towing a boat, while on 80 milligrams of OxyContin , but hey I am collecting a check, right? I was always the early driver; I love driving at 2:00 a.m., because I love to drive and I am good at keeping my people safe.

The fights that you have to go through with CRPS are things you do not even consider. It's not just the pain, its dealing with the lack of sleep and the emotional and mental issues that will rear their ugly heads as often as possible. If you have a family and kids as well, you have to figure out manage your whole life in a different way that doesn't need your sanity involved.

To me it became me versus the beast. I wake up not knowing what's going to be throbbing from day to day. I think the fact that I never know what I can do tomorrow is one of the most frustrating aspects of CRPS. One day you can be at a low pain level, at least in my case, and the next day you can wake up and you can move without the wind hurting.

My obvious CRPS symptoms started showing up when one day at physical therapy, they had me do these simple nerve glides. My arm was not happy, my elbow turned purple, and all my skin fell off in three days, This was the first weird hint that led to the discovery and diagnosis of my CRPS. The dermatologist had never seen anything like it, he was stumped, but said CRPS was definitely possible by the explanation and examination. Finally, someone has the next clue. That took about two months to heal. He gave me some cream and sent me on my way. I did not go back to therapy, and it never happened again.

I returned to pain management and explained what the Dermatologist said, and I finally was able to get a Stellate Ganglion block , because it's considered a diagnostic test. More on this later.

Like many others in the beginning, no doctors knew what is going on, and my CRPS seemed to be spreading and, now I had Fibromyalgia symptoms at the same time. I went to no less than nine doctors before I found a friend who was a nurse practitioner that would try an SGB, at a local pain management doctor and finally after many unsuccessful steroid blocks of my neck and upper back. After reading about the block, I asked my pain management doctor to please try it because I did have shoulder pain too and supposedly that can be treated with this block. Since it was a diagnostic test, they agreed to try thank goodness. They let me do that since even WC covers it.

So, I finally get my first Stellate Ganglion Block (SGB) and on the table while it was happening, my arm pain went away. I can't even describe how happy I was because I had pain relief. CRPS is not known as the suicide disease for no reason.

At this point, I had a positive outcome and was so happy I found something that WC would pay for. I forgot to mention that I had to go to work court to the commissioner to get the shots authorized. Up until this point IWIF had tried to deny any kind of treatments, besides the surgeries, and just thought I needed to go back to work.

So, the first Stellate Ganglion Block pain relief lasted 10-days, That was a start, I knew there was hope now. I had just bought a new house thinking

I was going back to work like nothing happened, Well this never happened. I had eight weeks to get better and I did not. Now, I am fighting WC. With a house payment, I had lost my housing because my boyfriend got into trouble for fishing, and went to jail, leaving his teenagers in charge of me. Meanwhile IWIF wants me back at work but there's no way. I can't sleep, I can't get comfortable, and I can't type or write with my right arm and I'm not good with my left. My job was physical also. How do I drive people around and run equipment and use computers and calculate important information? If I cannot think right my work cannot be trusted, you cannot work when you are tired, and in pain. You cannot work if you have no right arm, and your right hand.

If I did not have the co-workers and supervisors that I had throughout this whole process, I do not even know where I would be right now? I cannot stress that enough. If you have CRPS, and you do not have a network, find yourself one quick, or find me.

The lawyer I ended up needing to hire, was a peach. My doctors told me that I was not going to go back anytime soon, and IWIF wanted me back sooner. I went to IWIF court, again and my lawyer told me to do what WC told me to do, which was go back to work. My doctor had a note that said I cannot go back to work, so I saw the judge again, and I do not know which time this was the third, fourth, fifth , sixth or seventh time finally. I told her I was trying, the meds I was on, and I told her that they wouldn't let me go to any other doctor and they keep denying any care. I asked go to Johns Hopkins, and was approved but somehow, Johns Hopkins had some kind of note saying that I had some kind of bad drug habit which I have never failed a drug test except for marijuana, one time and I'll explain that in a bit. I did not want to take all the opioids they were prescribing; I think at

113

that time I was given three, 60 mg OxyContin a day, and I was in so much pain, I thought I wanted to die.

Sometimes it comes down to the lesser of two evils. At this time, they were evil, and I was not. When I told the judge what was going on, she told my case manager, and my lawyer to go out in the hall, and work it out. Well, in the hall it ended up I am not going back to work, and they ordered me to Johns Hopkins, which I never got to go to because that weed habit, they were claiming I had from Doctor Z, and my one failed drug test.
So, back to square one, I did not have to go back to work yet, and I did not get any more treatment. So, what do you do next? This is only about 20-months into my CRPS diagnosis, so you can see how much fun I have had. I had four months to go, before I would not be able to return to my job.

During this time, I had some doozies of a doctor, one was Doctor Z. I overheard him yelling at an 80-year-old woman in a wheelchair that she needed to stop crying before he could speak to her, and then he will come back when she calms down. Right then, I figured I was in trouble. He came in to talk to me, and basically told me I was faking, so that I can get money from WC. When I told him I was not, he said that I failed my urine test for marijuana, and I explained that I use marijuana instead of opioids as much as I can. So, he had me crying, and I said just let me go, I have to pick up my daughter at daycare. He then decided I was unable to pick up my daughter because I was having a mental break down because maybe the marijuana, not sure. He decided to call WC. and tell them that I was faking it, so I lost all my benefits, and I had no money. I just bought a house have not mentioned the house yet. I am lucky he did not call Child protective Services like he threatened to do that day. It was enough, I lost my income, and was all on my own after the boyfriend trouble.

114

At, this time my primary care doctor was able to prescribe my pain medications, and I was able to get my blocks at the Anne Arundel medical center. He was now prescribing my medications and knew what I was taking, and allowed the marijuana, because he is familiar with pain syndromes, as his wife has fibromyalgia. This was the start of me hitting my lawyer hard. He kept telling me just go to work, and do my job. I still could not use my right arm, and I could not sleep. I wanted to cut my arm off. At, this point we were waiting for our next hearing with the WC commissioner to get my money reinstated, and discuss the plan for me.

We finally, went to the commissioner and she thought that it was crazy to have me working on medication you cannot drive on. I got my payments back, therapy, and pain management too. This happened about five times, I had to keep going back every month, my nurse practitioner at IWIF did not think I needed anything but to work.

As per the commissioner, in one of these battles, I was supposed to be able to go to Johns Hopkins for a special pain management program. The commissioner ordered it to happen, so I was really excited. It took me probably 18-months to get to this point at this point the commissioner realized what my job was. When I called John's Hopkins to set up my appointment, I got a call back saying I was denied because WC said I had a substance abuse issue, thank you Doctor Z. The marijuana.

At this point, I'm ready for another Stellate ganglion block, I decided to switch doctors again. My next doctor was one I saw before the CRPS. They repeated the Cortisone shots in my neck and then burned my nerves. That did not work, and it definitely did not make anything better, it probably made things worse. After deciding that I could not stand this anymore, I started reading and reading. I found information on stellate ganglion blocks on Doctor HH's website: www.rsdrx.com. I think that man saved my life.

At the time, of this block, I had a bout of weird sweating that was unexplainable, on the arm I wanted to chew off. So, it's block time. Yay! I got the first block, and it was magical helped my arm stopped aching and no sweats, immediately. I could not believe it, But yes it didn't hurt very much at all anymore. That lasted 10-days, so I went back three weeks later, and they scheduled me for another one. The first block was a good sign, so they thought it would be a good idea to do another. I am not sure what happened, but after the first block, all of a sudden, my right leg started hurting, with sciatica really bad. This was out of the blue, I definitely did not do anything to hurt it. This was another mystery.

So, I go back to the pain management doctor and explain what happened and he said it was not possible so now I get a lumbar block for my leg that helped some for about 3 weeks , but it seemed like if I didn't sleep or I over did something, I would wake up and my leg would feel like my arm. At this point they tried Gabapentin, 3600 mg a day, and it did nothing, they tried Cymbalta, nothing, Lyrica, nothing, Everything they tried did not do anything. The only relief I had was the oxycodone, and I tried to take that as little as possible. I could not sneak in any marijuana or CBD because it showed up on the test once, I tried. I think I have tried everything you can possibly try.

So, now my arm was a dull roar not too horrible, but it definitely kept me from sleeping and working. That was a horrible nightmare. My legs were a pain in my butt literally. I would have a good-days, but I had more bad days at this point. I was still off work on temporary disability and running out of time, because WC was still fighting me instead of helping, and my lawyer

116

was worthless. All he did was keep telling me that I had to go back to work, then we have a hearing with the commissioner, and they would tell me I did not have to come back to work. We went back-and-forth like this a bunch, and the last time I was still waiting to go to Johns Hopkins. I have never messed up a drug test with anything other than marijuana, or CBD. Basically, the nurse case manager at WC, lied so I would not get treated at Johns Hopkins, period.

Then IWIF demanded an occupational evaluation. This was a complete joke. I received a letter saying that I would have to do a work evaluation with Some company that tests workers, where they see what work you can do. I was told they have to follow my doctor's orders, which at the time was no reaching, bending, stairs bearing weight, and limited to lifting five lbs. I showed up at 7:00 a.m., with a migraine, I was getting them four times a week. I had slept at my mother's house that night, so she could drive me because I still was not driving myself. I had migraines and a child to get to school, and the appointment was 7:00 a.m., Thanks mom! So, I show up, and told the nurse that I had a migraine, but I was able to keep going, and do the test, even if I had to stop and puke, which I did seven times. I did my best. That was the worst experience in my life. I have limited mobility in my hand and I am not allowed to lift over five pounds, they did not honor my doctor's orders, and made me climb steps which I am not allowed to do. I was forced to do multiple exercises I was not capable of, then they wanted me to walk a quarter-mile. At, this point because of my leg, I could barely walk because I tried the other tests I had to do. They forced me to do an exercise to screw in nuts and bolts over my head. I had to use my fingertips to pass, but I didn't know this. Since I cannot use my fingertips, I use the outside of my hands, and got it all done in no time. I thought I was good. In between all this, I am puking probably every 15 to 20 minutes from my migraines, and I do everything I can. At, the end the lady was not very nice, and she said thank you, and goodbye.

When my lawyer got the letter from the "therapy" place, it said that I was drunk, puking, and belligerent and I refused to do the tests. They never mentioned my "alleged migraine. If I am drunk, why didn't they tell me I was drunk at the start? Should I be tested drunk? What if I fell? I had no idea puking meant your actively drunk, but yet they did not say I was staggering, or slurring my speech or anything like that during the whole process. Surely, I would have smelled like drunk vomit, versus migraine dry heave vomit?

I know what a drunk smells like, I divorced one as soon as I smelled him like that, and my toddler brought me a baggie. I had enough to deal with besides a weak man who was hiding cocaine and alcohol issues. Why not tell me, so my mom could attest that I had no alcohol, or maybe call a police officer? Could I have gotten a breathalyzer? I swear on my life I was not drunk; I can assure you my mother would not be involved if she thought I had done anything wrong, she was also a non-believer in CRPS, but I had her help because I had a small child that matters most to both of us. I involved my mom at the time to be able to vouch for me, knowing if I was with her, she would know my every move , in case this sort of thing happened.

I did do all the tests that were not covered under my doctor's restrictions list, I may have completed them not according to directions, but I did them the only way I could because, I have no feeling in the tips. I dropped a bunch of nuts before I even got one in, the nurse saw me struggling, and I switched the way I held them, she never said I cannot, and put everyone I could in that board. To this day I cannot reach the height, as to what they

118

were trying to force me do. I had no idea that I had to do it exactly according to directions, or it is a total failure. I thought I just had to do it, to show them that I could get it done. If you do not think this gave me PTSD...who remembers these details 15-20 years later.

I found all this out a week later when my peach of a lawyer called and said now, if I do not go back, I can lose my insurance benefits. When my lawyer got this letter he said, Elisabeth this is not good, you are going to lose everything, you did not try, they think you are a drunk, and they want you at work because now, a drunk should be on pills driving five people in a van or a boat? Let's just say I was very scared. After this, Independent of the IWIF events, my employer requested I see the state medical examiner to review my case, and see if they can alter my job duties so I can at least try and do something, anything that does not require heavy machinery, lifting, sitting, or typing, you get the picture.

The heavens must have intervened with the timing on that letter requesting an independent evaluation. When I went to the Maryland State Medical Examiner, I was so nervous, I am not going to lie. I know I had plenty of documentation, and I couldn't stand up straight, due to my usual awful spasms. his office staff was so nice, no one was mean or scary, He was so very nice. He reviewed my x-rays, and my doctor's notes, and examined me. He agreed that there is not much that I can do that won't be painful and yes, I am messed up. With that I was fully released from duty . He saw the CRPS diagnosis, and everything. At, that moment I was free of worrying if I would have my next check. What a load off my mind. All that fighting with IWIF, for naught. Free in 45-minutes!

Since this was independent from WC insurance, I did not have to worry anymore, now my job was putting me out on permanent disability. Had they tried to treat me, I might have been able to work, had I received the proper care.

To this day, I wish I could sue IWIF, Doctor Z, whom I complained about, and my peach of a lawyer. I represented myself in the hearings, basically, because my lawyer did not read my medical reports, and I felt like even he thought I was faking, whenever he kept telling me do what they say. I loved my job so much, if I could have kept working, I would have. Being a field biologist is different than an office job, and I was no good in the office either. If it was not for the commissioner taking notice of my case, I do not think, I would be here today. The stress of that situation, knowing my lawyer thinks I am faking, and Doctor Z, calling in saying I was a fake, all the while they would not let me get any blocks.

My saving grace was having good health insurance, I said screw it, after my release from employment, and let them sort it out. That began my better treatment, because I was able to use my health insurance, because I never settled my IWIF case. I am not going to think about that until I have to.

Somewhere around this time both legs now ached horribly, and my arm was still waiting for a block. What the heck! So, I wait three weeks and see my anesthesiologist at the local hospital and he shrugs his shoulders. So, now what? He thinks about it and decides to do bi-lateral lumbar block, meanwhile my back and butt crack would not stop sweating.

My anesthesiologist suggested physical therapy at a local place connected to a pain management office. I am not sure what happened at physical therapy the first day I went, they had me do some simple nerve glide exercises and some very simple exercises ,like walk the wall with my fingers. Whatever happened in that session, I woke up the next

120

day, and my elbow was purple, bright purple not a bruise, and then all my skin fell off that I think was when they figured I have complex regional pain syndrome CRPS.

At, this point I was pretty fed up with my care. I had to do something different so I got online, and I started looking around for new treatments. I forget where I found her, but I found Doctor MC at George Washington University Hospital (GWU). She was recommended to be the local expert on CRPS, as George Washington University Hospital is a teaching hospital. They were doing a ketamine experiment, and I was able to sign up, though it was a nine month wait. During that waiting period she gave me a SGB block, and some lumbar blocks to hold me off until I was able to go to my Ketamine trial.

The ketamine infusion... When I went in for my infusion there were only two beds available and they were in the recovery room, where they were doing colonoscopies. If you had an infusion then you can imagine what it's like to hear farts, farts, and more farts while you are under ketamine. Lol! The atmosphere kind of made it hard to relax and do what you need to do but I was able to hide my head and listen to my favorite music and relax. The girl that walked in with me in the other bed walked in with a cane, and she told me she had horrible foot pain. The first day of infusion was interesting and it helped, When we both walked out, she did not need her cane. That was pretty amazing. When I left, I felt really good I think I was kind of loopy but I definitely felt like it knocked down a lot of the crazy stabbing pain, so two more days to go. The second day was fine. The foot girl next to me had a minor problem with snakes in her experience, and got very emotional. The nurses were not really able to handle her snakes , but I was able to talk to her and help her not see snakes. I was on a roller coaster, so we had snakes and roller coasters, Oh my! I think the worst part of the ketamine is having to pee. I learned to just get a diaper and deal

121

with it. They don't let you get up, and having to concentrate on not being "alive" can ruin the whole ketamine benefit if you cannot relax. Day two, I left and I felt pretty much like day one may be a little bit better. Went home and slept it off and went back the next day. This is when your driver will say yay! Last time! Do not forget to reward whomever has to bring you to the infusions. The final day went just like the second day, hopefully the ketamine stuck today. The most important thing with the infusion I think is to stay as relaxed as possible. I had no bad experiences had my diaper, peed when I wanted to, never broke my mellow. When we left on the last day, I was starving, as you cannot eat before and it was six or seven hours wait until food. I was hungry so we stopped to eat near GWU. The place we went to, our server stole my credit card number and by the time I got home there was $3,000 of charges for chocolate roses and heating oil on my card. That's always fun!

After the ketamine infusions, I felt better I was able to reduce my medicines and a half which was great. After about three months my back started bothering me again and I had to go look for blocks again, the wait for infusions at the time was up to 13-months.

After that I was just surviving on blocks, until one day my anesthesiologist told me that I had too many blocks and he could not give me any more so he sent me off to pain management for narcotics , except the pain management doctor thought the narcotics were making my pain so , no narcotics for me .... I ended up getting more blocks and finding medical marijuana, which was not legal yet, but I was desperate and getting suicidal again. I stuck with that doctor for six months, and found another doctor who could do Stellate blocks, but not very well. It wasn't worth the wait at GWU, or so I thought. The next doctor, did more blocks I am not supposed to have, but I was able to get narcotic relief again until I accidentally tested positive for marijuana and out, I went. So again, I had to find another doctor at this point. I found Choice Pain Management which has been my savior until this day. Doctor TS, and Doctor RS, they do the best blocks, and are willing to hunt down every nerve fiber, I loved the doctors there. I immediately he knew enough about CRPS, that I trusted him to take over my care. He wasn't trying to take all my pain medicines away and understood the pain levels that I could experience. He also was knowledgeable about SGBs, and done expertly. I have been going there for about five years, and I have been happy as I can be without having a Tampa spine center type facility in my area. I still need to find a specialist that can do something other than shots, maybe therapy, or something.

Handling daily life takes most of my energy, it is the same things I used to do, I do not understand why now it sucks and it is no fun, nothing changed, but everything. After I lost my job, I had to reevaluate my life. There's a reason they call CRPS the suicide disease. I think the mental stress of this disease is one of the harder parts to handle, especially when family and many doctors don't understand what we are experiencing on a daily basis. To this day, my mom still thinks I am a junkie, and I do not try hard, but she is not the one with aches, throbbing, stabbing, and cramping pains day, and night. It does not help I have advanced Degenerative Disc Disease (DDD), along with the CRPS. The doctors believe my case of CRPS is making my disc pain worse, causing all my spasms. I was supposed to get ketamine again, but due to a miscommunication, I had waited another nine months for naught. Talk about crushing! A week before my appointment, they cancelled my infusion because someone missed the note that I had completed my pre-check early, because I was headed out of town, and would not be able to check in normally, but I was coming on time. Since rescheduling would take at least another nine months if they let me back

123

in the program, and did not get mad I 'missed' my infusion. So, I gave up trying.

Currently, I alternate between several types of blocks, depending on what hurts the worst that month. I am able to achieve some pain relief from Stellate ganglion blocks, Medial Branch Blocks (MBB), and Lumbar Blocks (LB). For me, the SGB block was magical for those hard to explain CRPS symptoms, like the weird sweating, or unexplainable blood pressure or other oddities. I also was getting 30 trigger point injections a month,and then my pain doctor that does not do blocks but does my shots before he retired suddenly in October.

My future goal is to find a specialist that can treat me with the proper ketamine protocol including boosters and all the options available today. Where I will find that, I am not sure yet? I think I am Florida bound or Bust. Tampa is my next stop. I want to be one of the lucky folks that are ahead in this game of surviving.

TWENTY-FIVE YEARS LIVING WITH CRPS AND STILL GOING
Daryn Brown

In the summer of 1997, I had just graduated high school, and was getting ready to go off to college soon. Since I was a high school freshman, I knew I wanted to work in theater as a stage manager. I was so excited I had my first non-school-related stage management job at a local theater for the summer. It did not pay well, so I also got a job working as a server at a local restaurant. A few weeks into summer, I hurt my wrist. I went to the doctor, who took x-rays and determined it was a minor wrist sprain. She wrapped it with an ace wrap and told me to just rest it for a couple of weeks and it would be okay. I thought little about it and continued working my busy schedule that usually involved working as a server in the morning, then going to the theater for rehearsals. It didn't take long before I realized the pain was getting worse and not better in my wrist. At first, I tried to ignore the worsening pain, but it quickly became unbearable, so I went back to the doctor. She did more x-rays that showed nothing, so she sent me to a hand therapist. By this time, my hand had clenched tightly in a fist. The skin was shiny, there was a little swelling, and the pain and hypersensitivity were like nothing I had ever experienced before.

The hand therapist listened to my symptoms, and only needed one look to determine that she thought I had reflex sympathetic dystrophy (RSD), which is now known as complex regional pain syndrome (CRPS). She referred me to a pain management doctor, and I made an appointment. Unlike most people, I had heard of CRPS before, and knew a little about it, as my paternal grandmother had it. I could get into the pain doctor quickly, and he agreed with the hand therapist I had CRPS. All the research suggests it's more likely to have success and even remission, the sooner a diagnosis is made, and treated. They diagnosed me within three months, and I

125

started nerve blocks immediately. I had no way of knowing at this point how much CRPS was going to impact the rest of my life. I had several stellate ganglion nerve blocks over the next few weeks. Though they helped for a couple of days to a couple of hours, we knew I was going to have to try other things. I worked with the hand therapist a lot and my doctors put me on gabapentin and Topamax to help get things to calm down. To my relief, we were able to get it under control by the time I left for college, or so I thought. The first few years of having CRPS, it remained very localized to my left arm from below the elbow through my hand.

When the pain flared up, it was excruciating. I remember I was with my parents somewhere, and I felt like I was being stabbed in the arm with a knife that was on fire. I kept looking to see if there was something on me when I finally found an eyelash, one of my eyelashes. I got it off my arm, but could not believe that such a small thing could cause so much pain. When I was not flared up though, I had no pain, and you would never know anything was wrong. In 1999, I flared up and could not get it under control for a few months. My doctor, who I trusted a lot, suggested getting a spinal cord stimulator (SCS) implanted. After doing a lot of research and talking to my parents, we did the trial. I scheduled it, and planned to stay with my parents for the few days of the trial. My doctor placed the leads in my back, and secured the battery pack to the outside of my body for the trial. It seemed to work pretty well, so I went through with getting a permanent SCS. I was very sore after the surgery but could not wait to go back to college with my friends. I was also the stage manager for Peter Pan, which was currently in rehearsal, and I resolved to finish the show. My amazing roommate at the time helped bandage my scars and monitor them, as one was in the middle of my spine, just below my shoulder blades, and the other was just above my butt on the right side. I will never forget late one night when we got home from a friend's house. My roommate went to do the usual bandage change, and said she thought she could see some of the battery poking out. I got scared and did not know what was going on. I called my parents, and told them what my roommate saw. We all decided that my roommate, and another friend would drive me the hour and a half to the ER nearest to my parents, who met us there.

When my doctor finally arrived, he said the battery had floated to the surface, and was pushing out of my body. He had seen nothing like it! (There were two places where it looked like the skin had worn away and the silver battery was actually poking out of my skin.) He decided he would reimplant the battery on the other side of my lower back. I stayed at my parents' house for a couple of days while I recovered. I turned twenty-one while I was recovering at my parents' home. Many people like to do something memorable for their 21st birthday, and mine was certainly memorable. We had a nice dinner at one of my favorite restaurants, and because it was my 21st birthday, my parents let me order a glass of wine. I was still very sore from the surgery, but dinner was going well, and it was nice to be able to do something "normal". I got up to go to the bathroom toward the end of the meal when my mom stopped me. I was wearing light khaki pants and a button-down shirt tucked in. when my mom saw my back, she got scared. My entire back and hips were covered in blood and fluid. Afraid that this battery was pushing itself out of my body again, my dad quickly paid the bill, and we headed to the nearest emergency room. Just the place I wanted to be on my big birthday.

When we got to the ER, the doctors looked at my back and told me the battery was not pushing out, but some of the stitches had popped, and the incision needed to be re-stitched. I was so relieved that was all it was and, after stitching it and cleaning it up, I was ready to go. Though I was still sore from the surgery, I was ready to go back to school. I could not wait to

127

get back to stage managing Peter Pan, which was nearly ready for tech rehearsals. Tech rehearsals are always intense, as it is when all aspects of the show (e.g., acting, scenery, lighting, sound, etc.) are first combined. As the stage manager, I was responsible for running these rehearsals and learning from the director and designers when to call cues to change the lights and sound. I remember sitting in the theater with a pillow behind my back and friends bringing me an ice pack occasionally to help with the post-surgical pain and swelling. I had pain medication to help with the pain but did not want to take it while I was working because it made me tired and fuzzy headed. Looking back, I do not know why I was so resolved to finish this show as the stage manager, though I could have stepped down easily. A friend of mine covered rehearsals while I was out, and could have done the whole thing, but I insisted I had to do it. At the time, the things that were most important to me were my friends and theater.

Unfortunately, shortly after the show closed my SCS started pushing itself out again. This time, both the battery in my lower back, and the device between my shoulder blades were visible. I asked my doctor to remove the whole thing. The SCS had helped a little, but my doctor could not figure out why it kept pushing out of my body, and more importantly, how to stop it from doing so. Flare-ups continued to come and go, but I learned to not let them stop me from doing the things I wanted to do. I even went to work in Scotland for a couple of months between my junior, and senior years. After college, I was accepted into an intern program at the McCarter Theatre in Princeton, NJ. I was so excited and could not wait to get there. I knew it would be hard, but I also knew it would give me the experience and connections needed to pursue my dream of stage managing in NYC. After my nine-month internship, I moved to NYC. I met a lighting designer on a show at McCarter, and we started to date. He already lived in NYC, so we got an apartment together. Life was going even better than I expected.

My boyfriend seemed perfect for me. My friends were amazing. I had the best and most supportive family, and I was working my dream job in the city I loved. Who could ask for anything more? I found a wonderful doctor in NYC who worked with me to control my flare-ups. I don't remember exactly when, but during my first few years in NYC, the CRPS spread up my left arm and through my right arm and hand. My flare-ups also got harder and harder to get back under control. My doctor tried every type of medication he could think of over the years. At some point, we figured out that if we could get my hand to open, the flare would calm down. There was a time he would try to put me to sleep with propofol and pry my hand open. I would wake up minutes later with a random object in my hand, trying to keep it open.

Unfortunately, it did not work well, and the object would either pop out of my hand as it fought the clench or my hand would tighten around the object, getting it stuck in my hand. When it got stuck in my hand, he would again have to use the propofol to remove the object. In 2008, during a particularly difficult flare that we could not get under control, my doctor, and I talked about the benefits and risks of implanting a pump in my body to consistently deliver baclofen to my spine. I was already on the highest dose of oral baclofen, which had initially worked well, but my body kept adjusting to it, causing me to need to keep increasing the dose. Oral baclofen has a lot of potential side effects and the higher the dose I took, the worse the side effects could get.

Eventually, when I reached a dose that worked for me, it caused too many side effects. Because an internal pump could deliver a much higher dose of baclofen without causing adverse side effects, we proceeded with a trial. Where he injected baclofen directly into my body, into the area where it was most effective. The trial was successful, and in 2008, we decided to proceed with surgery to implant the pump. By then, I always had some level of pain in my hands and arms, and it became much worse during a flare-up. In addition to infusing the baclofen through the implanted pump, my doctor tried adding morphine, dilaudid and several other pain medications in an effort to obtain relief. Eventually, we decided to use the baclofen alone, as it was the most helpful to me.

Over the next few years, I lived a fairly normal life. I took a break from theater, and began working in event technology at a hotel. After a couple of years, the hotel sold my department to a third party. I decided not to interview with the new company, and instead found a similar job in a different hotel. I still had occasional break-thru flares, but usually, if we turned the pump up a bit, the flare-up would calm down. Soon, however, I had a few more stubborn flares that would not respond to increasing the rate of my pump. As the effectiveness of the baclofen pump waned, we continued to seek other viable treatments. Eventually, we tried some low-dose ketamine infusions, which did not seem to help. I also shifted to using lyrica instead of gabapentin to see if it would make a difference-it did not, and then, I tried several antidepressants, none of which provided relief, or otherwise helped me. Eventually, I got tired of taking so many medications that did not seem to help, so I stopped all medication, except oral pain medication, as needed and the baclofen in my pump.

In February 2010, everything changed. I had just left work, and was walking to the subway, taking my usual route. It was a 15-minute walk to the subway, so I would often call my parents, or a friend to say hi on my walk. On February 27, 2010, I was talking to my mom as I approached an intersection. I noted the light signaled that I had the right of way to cross the street, so I did. The next thing I remember was telling my mom I had to go as I was just hit by a car. I did not learn until much later that I had not actually hung up, and disconnected the call, and my poor mom could hear all the surrounding commotion. Being several states away, and unable to do anything helpful, I knew how hard and traumatizing it was for my mom. I remember a bunch of people crowding around to make sure I was okay. Someone must have called 911, and an ambulance took me to the hospital. I have almost no memory of the night. My mom called my boyfriend, who met me at the hospital.

Fortunately, the car that hit me was not going fast, and I did not break any bones or have any other major injury. I could go home that night after being checked out at the hospital. Though I did not have any new physical injuries, both of my hands flared up, and clenched tightly closed. I went to see my pain doctor, who promptly got to work trying to get the flare under control. He turned my baclofen pump up, and increased my lyrica. Unlike other times, however, these interventions did not help to calm the flare at all. After a few more days, I started having horrible pain in my lower back and abdomen. My doctor sent me for x-rays to make sure he was not missing anything, and as a result, he discovered the catheter implanted in my spine, which was connected to the baclofen pump, had broken and become dislodged because the car knocked me down. This meant that the baclofen, including all the increases and boluses we had tried, were just spraying baclofen throughout my body, rather than directly into my spine. My doctor immediately scheduled me for surgery to repair the connection. In the meantime, my legs started causing me new problems. I began having trouble walking, and started using a cane to get around. I also had much more pain in my legs, similar to the pain I had in my hands.

My doctor tried everything he could think of. They even admitted me to the hospital for a high-dose round of ketamine. The low-dose ketamine never helped, but my doctor wanted to see if a much higher dose would do so. In the hospital, they gave me an extremely high dose of ketamine for five straight days. Not only did the treatment not help, but it caused me terrible hallucinations that would continue for many weeks after the treatment. The hallucinations were very scary. I had been home from the ketamine infusion admission for about a day when my boyfriend left to do some work for a couple of hours. I was sitting on the couch resting and watching TV, and I must have fallen asleep. Next thing I know, I woke up to a loud pounding on the door. Apparently, I hallucinated that people were coming to get me. (It was always the same hallucination). In my, confused state, I pushed all our furniture to barricade the door, and put the chain on the door. My boyfriend got home and could not get in. He had no idea what was going on. Ketamine had not helped my pain, and the scary hallucinations meant that the only time I would now use ketamine was during surgery. Doctors believe the ketamine would help prevent the CRPS from continuing to spread throughout the rest of my body.

I also tried lidocaine infusions, several types of nerve blocks, and several new medications. Nothing was helping, and my health was continuing to decline. I ended up getting fired from my last job because they said I was not at 100% capacity. This was such a stressful and scary time for me. I was having the biggest spread of my CRPS ever, and I was in so much more pain. I pursued two lawsuits - one against the driver of the car that knocked me down and another against my employer for wrongfully firing me. Not only was I far away from my family, but my boyfriend had completely shut down and became unable to cope with any of it. Somehow, he also broke his foot and was using crutches. My parents and I decided it made sense for me to fly back home to Columbus for a four-week admission to an inpatient rehab center called Dodd Hall, which was part of The Ohio State University Wexner Medical Center (OSUWMC). I was not thinking long term; All I could focus on was whether I was going to this intense program.

My next step would depend on how well this program went. I quickly packed what I needed for the program and flew home to Columbus. As expected, the program was quite rigorous. I did PT
and OT every day, along with some counseling.

About halfway through the program, I knew I could not go back to NYC, and needed to be with my parents, sister, and nephews. I called my boyfriend, and told him. His response was to ask how to get all my stuff to me. Obviously, that meant he was not even considering coming to Columbus, and after ten years together, our relationship was over. I was neither sad, nor relieved, I felt nothing. I kept expecting, and waiting for sadness, but it never happened. We talked a few times after that, but there was nothing there. In hindsight, our relationship should have ended much sooner than it did, but it was now over.

The Dodd Hall program was very helpful, but my legs had gotten much worse. I was using a walker to get around and still could not get far. So, once again, I started working with some new doctors, who tested me for everything and anything they could think of to make sure we were not missing anything. While I did learn that I had small fiber neuropathy and some other minor issues, the CRPS was the real problem. My doctors were wonderful and willing to try anything to help get my pain level under control. We tried more ketamine and lidocaine infusions, along with various other medications and nerve blocks. We tried adding several other pain medications through my pump, and many other things. I even tried another SCS, only after lots of allergy testing to make sure that was not the reason my body rejected the old ones. As usual, the new SCS did not help, and it did not stay in long. Nothing ever touched the pain.

Since I had left Dodd Hall, I was living with my parents in their two-bedroom condominium. In 2011, I was standing in my bedroom with my walker when my legs seemed to collapse out of nowhere. I did not fall hard, and I fell on a carpeted floor, but I still managed to break both the tibia and fibula on my right leg. I had surgery to implant a rod in my leg. I was home recovering for a couple of days when the rod somehow broke. They took it out and put another rod in. Unfortunately, that rod also broke after a few days. Finally, they decided to do plates and screws in my leg. I had an external fixator and was wheelchair-bound while it healed. When it was finally healed, I resumed PT to work my way out of my wheelchair. It was incredibly challenging and a lot of work, but I was so eager to be able to walk again. I progressed and thought I was done with the wheelchair for good. I developed a drop foot in my left foot, and I was sent to a podiatrist who fitted me for a brace to help. However, because my skin was so sensitive, I was not able to wear it. I worked on the drop foot a lot in PT, and eventually, it did go away. A brief time later, I developed a contracture in my right foot that caused it to rotate. It made walking even more difficult. Unfortunately, as my pain increased, I returned to the wheelchair, as walking was intolerable.

I continued working on PT. I was always in a lot of pain but was figuring out what I could and could not do. I was reconnecting with friends from high school, and college who lived in Columbus, and I was making new friends. I felt like I might have a life again. Then in 2012, my family was supposed to go to Cleveland to see the rest of my family. I was not feeling good, so my mom stayed back with me. The next part, I have no memory of just what others have told me and the medical notes in my chart. I guess I was having trouble breathing and something did not seem right with me. I was lethargic and becoming incoherent, so my mom took me to the emergency room. Things progressed quickly when I got there, and I ended up on a

134

ventilator and life support. They told my parents I developed ARDS (acute respiratory distress syndrome). I was on the vent for a couple of weeks. They tried to get me off it a few times but were not able to do so. Eventually, they were able to wean me off. I ended up at another rehab center (Wexner Heritage) while I got my strength back before going home.

While at Wexner Heritage, I met one of the most amazing people I have ever met. Lori taught me about Reiki and Urban Zen. I had never heard of either. She worked with me as often as she could using essential oils and teaching me how to relax. She continued to work with me when I got home, and is still the only person to be able to get me to a place where she can touch my legs without me jumping out of my skin. She also introduced me to some other amazing people who taught me about Laughter Yoga and Zentangle. These things helped keep my spirits up, and allowed me to keep fighting, though they did not do much to decrease the actual pain.

I was not home long when I had to go back to the hospital after I developed respiratory syncytial virus (RSV), which is another respiratory illness usually found in babies and kids. Luckily, I was there for only a few weeks, and soon I was able to return home.

In 2014, after doing a lot of research and talking to doctors, my dad drove me to Cleveland to see a doctor at Cleveland Clinic. Doctor S-H, was well known for his work with CRPS, he had also been my grandma's doctor many years ago. He was going to try Prialt (a synthetic Cone Snail venom) in my pump to see if it worked. If it did, he would give the needed info to my doctors in Columbus to maintain it as none of them had used this medication. I had to be there for a couple of weeks while he slowly titrated the medicine up in my pump. While I was there, I stayed with my aunt and uncles. They all took such loving care of me, and my aunt taught me to

135

make beaded jewelry which has become a very relaxing hobby of mine. Once Doctor S-H, got the medication to a certain level, I was allowed to go back home to Columbus to see how it helped for a bit.

Again, I do not remember much from this time. It did not take long before I started acting unlike myself. My parents said I got incredibly angry and aggressive. I was fighting and hitting my dad. My dad said I got super strong, and it was exceedingly difficult to control me. I was also having horrible and terrifying hallucinations. My parents became concerned and took me to the ER. I was having a bad reaction to the Prialt. I had to be put on life support again while they removed the medication from my pump. They also had to restrain me to the bed. I guess I had pulled out my IV, and anything else connected to me. I do remember waking up at one point and realized I was tied down to a bed and got scared. I did not know I was in the hospital.

I finally got out of the hospital, and decided to focus on non-medical things like Urban Zen, Reiki, Laughter Yoga, and PT. I got stronger and more stable over time. I decided I was ready to try to go back to work part-time. I missed working in the theater so much as it was a huge part of my life for so long, and I missed feeling productive at work. I was fortunate that there are several good theater companies near me. I talked to one of them who decided they would love to have me part-time to assist the operations manager with things. I was so excited to be back in the theater again and the people there are amazing. Not only are they some of the most talented people I have ever met but some of the nicest and most caring people. As I could not drive, and I was still learning to get around in a wheelchair I learned how to take the bus near me to work. It was such a good feeling to have some of my independence back and I was feeling more like myself than I had in years. Having my independence and doing as much as I can myself has always been important to me and was even more important now. I built up my strength by pushing myself in my wheelchair over time. You have no idea how much strength and endurance it takes to get around in a wheelchair until you must do it. I was only working part-time and was always exhausted at the end of the day, but I felt like I had purpose again. I was also going out with friends a lot, as I had reconnected with some high school and college friends who lived nearby, and I made new friends.

One of my doctors finally had a new idea that was worth a try. He implanted an epidural in my back which was connected to an external pump that delivered bupivacaine (a numbing agent) directly, and consistently into my spine. Though this medication did not help the pain, it did help numb my legs, reducing the hypersensitivity. I was able to get pants and shoes on for the first time in years. Having the sensitivity under control made a dramatic difference in what I could do. I was much less worried about every gust of wind or person bumping me. I had a nurse who would see me at home once a week to change the needle that went into the port that was implanted. Initially, it was only supposed to be in for five days, but because it was working so well, my doctor let me keep it if it didn't cause more problems than it helped. However, I did have one negative effect, though we still are not sure if it was caused by the bupivacaine or the CRPS. I started developing large sores all over my legs. They would start as big water blisters, and they always seemed to open. With the bupivacaine running, I could not feel them at all and was able to treat them. My doctor sent me to a wound care specialist, who biopsied the sores to make sure they were not something else, and he determined that they weren't infected. His office staff gave me a topical ointment to put on the sores and showed me how to bandage them. I had no improvement, so after a couple of weeks they decided to try a different topical. I must have tried five or six distinct kinds of topicals and many different bandages and dressings.

Finally, I tried one called Silvercel (antimicrobial wound dressing), which was a cloth-like square covered in little silver dots. You could cut off the size you needed, get it damp, put it on the wound, and tape it down. Though I had tried other products containing silver without success, this one worked. Nevertheless, I still healed very slowly, and was left with huge scars all over my legs.

Though I was still in a lot of pain I had learned some ways to cope with it and for the first time since the car hit me, I felt like I was living life rather than just watching life go on around me. My parents and I also started talking about the possibility of me moving out to my own place. We found an apartment building less than a half a mile away from my parents' place. It had just started construction and in an early stage when we started talking to the developers. They were willing to build out a unit that was fully wheelchair accessible and specifically built for my needs. Of course, it was more than I could have ever expected. The apartment was perfect. I was one of the first people to move into the building in 2015, when it was done. I quickly made friends with some of the other people living in the building, and I was enjoying living on my own for the first time in my life. My friends started to ask me about dating, and meeting someone new, now that I was able to get out more. Honestly, since my relationship had ended when I first moved back to Columbus, I had not given relationships much thought. When I was in, and out of hospitals, and continuously having serious medical issues, it was the furthest thought in my head. Now that I was stable, all I could think about was who would want to get involved, by choice, with the medical mess that was my life. My friends finally convinced me to try online dating. I had never done, or thought much about it before all of this, as I was in a relationship for ten years. They persisted, and I signed up. My profile picture was a full body of me in my wheelchair, and I mentioned a little about my CRPS in my profile. I figured I would rather be upfront, and honest, thinking I was protecting myself from getting hurt. Though in some ways it should not matter, I did not want to talk to someone, and be interested, and only when we decided to meet, they would pull up, and unexpectedly find that I used a wheelchair. I have never been a big dater. I did not date in high school, or college, and then I met someone who I was with until the car injured me, so I was shocked at the number of replies I got. Most people commented that they appreciated the upfront honesty, and it was fun to meet people who I was unlikely never to ever meet.

Things were going well, given the circumstances. I had started to get more serious with one of the guys, Gary, who I had met online, and he was often at my apartment. I started having problems with my epidural, and the pump kept malfunctioning. At first, it would run for a few hours then start beeping at me, and within a day or so, it was beeping constantly. Of course, because the pump did not work, medication was not getting delivered into my spine at all. I called my doctor who had me come right in. After playing around with the pump for a bit, while I was getting x-rays done, he determined there was a kink in my implanted epidural line and the port the needle went into had rotated. This surely meant more surgery to fix it. Fortunately, my doctor was able to get me into an operating room quickly, and he was able to do the necessary repair, sending me home that same night. My home health nurse returned the next day, and she got the pump running again. Everything seemed to return to how they were before the pump started acting up.

I had a good routine at work, and I loved being back in the theater, even if it was in a quite different role than in the past. I had built up my stamina, and was able to do much more before reaching my limit. I was at home with Gary, when I started to have a band of pain around my lower back and abdomen. It felt quite different than anything I had experienced in the past, and I had no idea what was going on. The pain kept getting worse to the point that I couldn't move. I had also become lethargic and spacey, and both my hands and arms were hurting, and starting to close. I called my parents, and we quickly decided that I needed another trip to the ER because something was not right. Once again, I have no memory of what followed, except what I was told later. Gary somehow got me in the car and took me to the ER. My doctor was paged, and he quickly came down to examine me. It appeared that my pump had again malfunctioned, and this time, the result was that I was in serious baclofen withdrawal, which could be deadly.

I ended up on life support for several weeks, while they removed the pump entirely, and got my body back under control. When I woke up, I was shocked to see Gary there, and even more shocked when I heard how long I had been on life support, and how often he was there. He had bought me a stuffed dog wearing an OSU shirt to watch over me when he had to go to work. It was so sweet. He had also gotten to know my parents a little, even helping my dad address envelopes for his campaign. They needed my body to heal a lot more before they re-implanted another pump, but I could not be without the pump either. My team of doctors figured out a way to send me home for a while with the pump catheter implanted normally and the pump left outside my body, taped down to my abdomen. I had to be incredibly careful while it was attached that way. Because I was still in severe pain throughout my body, I would not be moving much anyway. I could not lay down to sleep, so I started sleeping in my living room in my armchair with an ottoman. Gary, who had moved in by this time, did not want to be far from me, so he started sleeping on the couch. I needed help doing nearly everything, as it was so difficult and painful to move. I could not get to the bathroom easily, so he would bring my commode close by, and he would help me transfer to and from it. When my medical team decided my body had healed adequately, my doctor brought me back into surgery and re-implanted the pump properly. Luckily, it was an outpatient surgery, and compared to everything else I had just been through, it was relatively easy. I was hospitalized for over a month because of the pump malfunction, and in many ways, I feel like I never fully recovered from everything that happened.

I was finally doing a lot better, and I even returned to work as I was able. Gary, and I were enjoying time together, and getting to know each other better. We had talked about getting a dog for a long time, and decided to start looking seriously. I never had a dog, but we had spent a lot of time with his aunt and uncle, who had two Pomeranians. When we would visit them, the dogs would always climb onto my lap to get loved on. It was the strangest experience, as these dogs did not hurt my legs at all. When even a hair from my head falling on my legs or a light breeze touches them, it is very painful, but the dogs did not hurt my legs at all. We had narrowed the breeds we were looking at, and Gary had responded to some ads regarding rehoming pets. While we were waiting to hear back, he found another listing that looked interesting, so we sent an email. The lister replied quickly, and we decided to meet them and the dog in person. On the way to meet them, we talked that if she were not afraid of my wheelchair, like some dogs are, and if she seemed to take to us okay, we would get her. She was even cuter in person than in the picture they had posted. She jumped right into my arms, and I knew she was ours. I did try to hand her back at one point, but she was not going. She decided she wanted to be with us. She sat on my lap on the short drive home, and I looked at the paperwork they gave us for her. It said she was an Olde English Bulldog, and listed her birthday as February 27th. That is the date of the accident that aggravated my CRPS, and added many more recent problems. I knew this dog was meant to be with us, and we named her Gemma. She has brought us so much love and laughter, I cannot, and do not want to imagine life without her.

The whole ordeal with the pump malfunctions had taken a lot out of me, and I was hoping nothing else would come up for a bit. I was wrong, a couple of months later I thought that I may have pulled a muscle or something. My mom had given me her little leg exercise machine to try and strengthen my legs. I had just started using it, and I soon realized that I had overdone it. When the pain kept getting worse, and I could barely move, we knew it was time for yet another visit to the ER. I could not even move enough for Gary to help me into a car, and we ended up calling an ambulance. After a very extensive exam, and many tests, they concluded I had developed an infection in the epidural space. They had to remove the implanted catheter and cut out and clean up a lot of the infected tissue in my lower back. Because they had removed so much tissue, they did not want to close me up until they were 100% certain they got all the infected tissue out. They sent me home with a wound VAC, and IV antibiotics. My home health nurse would come every week to change the wound VAC, and make sure everything was healing well. Once they were sure I was free of infection they finished closing me back up. However, I was now again without my epidural. My hypersensitivity was as bad as ever, and I realized how much the epidural had helped.

Once all my wounds were completely healed, I started doing warm water therapy. I tend to flare up doing anything much physical on land, but in the warm water my pain went down, and I could do a lot more. I was not able to stand for more than a couple of seconds on land, but in the water, I could stand for up to ten minutes. Not only that, but I was working on both building strength, and endurance and trying to desensitize to reduce my pain. Therapy was going well; except I did not get along well with my therapist. He had never worked with anyone with CRPS, and would simply tell me just to push through the pain. He kept trying to get me to do things on land that I knew would cause me problems. In the past, I would continue PT until insurance said they would not pay for more. Usually, the first couple times when insurance says I am out of PT days, the therapist tells them we are making progress and asks to extend my benefits, and they would often do so. I was hoping this would be the case again, and I was still trying to find a warm water pool near me that I could use on my own. Unfortunately, he decided he did not want to work with me anymore, and he discharged me.

In 2018, my doctor finally decided it was worth trying to re-implant another epidural, as it has been the only thing, I have done that has made much of a difference. It was another outpatient surgery, and my home nurse came two days later to connect the bupivacaine to my port. She was not able to get the needle in, and she did not understand why inserting the needle was problematic. We decided to give me a few more days to heal. She came back early the next week, and this time she was able to insert the needle into the port much more easily. As a result, I was re-connected to the bupivacaine. Unfortunately, it did not seem to work as well this time. For example, I would have to turn the pump up quite high to get any numbing feeling. My doctor believes that with all the damage that had been done to my lower back from the infection and its treatment was preventing the medicine from reaching the places it needed to reach to be helpful. After a few months, we decided to stop and remove the epidural.

In 2019, I thought I had caught a bug, as I had a fever, headache, and was throwing up. At first, I thought it would just go away on its own, and I was doing what I could to try and stay comfortable. When I was getting worse and not better, I knew I had to call my doctor, and let him know. He was concerned that I might have another infection, so he urged me to go to the hospital. The hospital ran lots of tests to try and figure out what was going on. I was far more coherent, and alert than I had ever before been in a hospital, which made this stay worse for me. In the first room I was in, I found a pile of ants on the ground. I told a nurse about it, and at first, she used a Clorox wipe to clean up the ant pile and throw them away. Then, she realized there were many more ants, and she needed to change my room. For assorted reasons, I changed rooms three, or four more times during the three weeks I was there. The other thing that made this hospitalization hard was that my dad was in the same hospital. He had been sick for a while, and it had gotten much worse. Also, he had suddenly lost a ton of weight. He had had throat cancer a few years earlier, and after radiation treatment he was cancer-free, but this was something entirely different.

Eventually, after ruling out other conditions, his doctors diagnosed him with severe pneumonia. So, my mom was visiting the hospital a lot, going back, and forth between our rooms. My doctors still could not figure out what was wrong with me, and they wanted to do an MRI. The problem with that was, despite the removal of the several implanted SCSs, I still had some metal in my back. The remaining metal, such as wires, had to be completely removed to do an MRI safely. Just as I was getting ready to go to surgery, they wheeled my dad in to see me. It was so good to see him, even if he had to wear a mask and gown. In surgery, the metal was removed so we could proceed with the imaging. The MRI provided my doctors a clean picture, and I was finally discharged to go home.

The last couple of years I have not had anything major come up, and fortunately, I have not had to be hospitalized again. However, my pain level has continued to increase, and my legs have become more sensitive than ever. In the past, I have always had to keep my legs elevated. I had custom wheelchair legs made that gave me more support when my legs were elevated. I always kept my legs up because I could not tolerate them being down. Now the increased pain and sensitivity prevents me from elevating them, as the back of my legs was unable to touch anything. I have tried to go back to work a few times, but I am not currently able to do that because it always causes intensified flares and extensive brain fog. Gary, and I have now been together for six years, and I cannot imagine a better partner to have at my side. He keeps me laughing and would do anything for me, if I thought it would help. Gary, and I moved just over a year ago to a condominium unit in the same building as my parents. We could not have timed our move any better either, as we got in, and settled just before the COVID-19 lockdown had started. We now have a lot more room, and everything is laid out better for us than in the apartment. And, as a bonus, we have a nice little porch that we love sitting on, especially in the evenings. Gemma loves the park behind our building, and she has made lots of dog buddies there. I was vaccinated for COVID in May, and unfortunately, it triggered the worst flare I have had in years. I had stopped getting flu shots many years ago, as I would always have a flare-up right afterward. A flare-up was, of course, a possibility with the COVID vaccine, but it was one that I needed to do, knowing that I would not do well with a COVID infection. It is now about six months since this flare began, and it shows no sign of calming down. Also, following the vaccination, I had a return of the awful swelling and sores all over my legs, which had been gone for years. I learned that I was right about the sores being very painful without the epidural.

145

Unfortunately, there are few treatments, or medications left for me to try, and for some of those few, such as Calmare therapy, I have found no doctor who uses it near me. I did try an infusion of, which is a bisphosphonate, which did nothing to help. A few weeks ago, I tried another infusion of pamidronate, which is another bisphosphonate now used more often than Reclast (zoledronic acid). So far, I have not noticed any improvement, but it has only been a few weeks. To notice any change can take up to six months. Italy has done a lot of promising research on a bisphosphonate called Neridronate that is administered by infusion However, the medication is not available in the U.S. for treatment of CRPS.

In many ways, I am frustrated that there are no other options for me to try right now. With this continuing flare, I am in too much pain to do much of anything, but I also know how lucky I am. I have the most amazing parents, and family, who have been right by my side fighting with me (and for me when I am unable to fight). I managed to meet an amazing guy who somehow can still see me beyond the disease, despite all the medical crap that can get in the way. We have the sweetest, most loving dog ever, and though I have lost some friends I have managed to hang on to some incredible friends. CRPS has taken a lot from me over the years, especially the past ten but I try to remain optimistic that they will learn more about CRPS, and be able to come up with more effective treatments.

Unfortunately, until they learn more about the disease, and how it works, they can only treat symptoms and we all have different symptoms that respond differently to treatments. My hope, and wish is that one day they will figure out how to effectively treat CRPS better, and people would not have to suffer in pain. In the meantime, I will keep fighting.

RISING FROM THE ASHES OF CRPS
Debbie Hall

My journey began in the spring of 2009. I was 41-years-old, a wife, and a mom. I was a special education teacher with a master's degree, and had been teaching for only six years. I had found my purpose life; to help children like my son who have learning disabilities, and other issues with learning, and behavior.

One night I was climbing into bed, and rolled my ankle as I got in, and sprained it. I could not believe that just climbing into bed could result in spraining my right ankle, but it did. It was not the first time, or the last time I sprained that ankle.

This time however was so very different. The pain was worse and the burning and buzzing I felt was strange and annoying. I could not keep my ankle still. It felt like ants were crawling all over me and I had to keep moving it.

I went to the orthopedic doctor and got an X-ray. "It is just sprained" the doctor said. Keep it wrapped up, and here are some crutches to use for a while, so you can stay off of it until it heals. The problem was it was not healing. It was getting worse. My ankle, foot, and lower part of my leg were swelling up even more, and were turning redder, and becoming splotchy. The doctor said to keep it elevated, and stay off of it. The thing was I was staying off of it. Then at my next appointment I told him it was now sensitive to anything touching it.

My primary doctor sent me to a neurologist to see if she could figure out what was going on. She did the nerve conduction study called an Electromyography (EMG). That was not fun at all! It was very painful, and I almost threw up on the doctor. All she could say is there is no nerve damage. She said, "I am sorry but I have no idea what is going on with you. I was sure nerve damage was going to show up on you. You have a lot of those symptoms."

I went to physical therapy, and within minutes as soon as I got nauseous the physical therapist knew exactly what I had. She said, "sorry, you have complex regional pain syndrome (CRPS) formally known as reflex sympathetic dystrophy (RSD). You need to go back to your orthopedic doctor, and tell him you have CRPS."

What baffled me next was that the orthopedic doctor actually said, "Why didn't I think of that?" He told me to go look it up online, that he is an orthopedic doctor, and does not deal with CRPS. I asked what doctor did deal with CRPS. He said," I have no idea. Go look it up online." Then he walked out of the room. That was the end of that except for physical therapy (PT).

Months had already gone by from the initial injury to this point. I was wearing a boot to keep me from moving my ankle around which felt very necessary to me, because the sensations of buzzing and ants made me feel like I had to move my ankle and foot all the time.

I researched CRPS, and found what we all find when we research it. That it is a rare disease with no known cure, and not much understanding as to why it happens to people. I was devasted. I thought this cannot be true. There has to be a doctor that knows about this, and how to treat it. That's when I found Doctor AK, at the International Research Foundation for RSD/CRPS. The best part was this was in the town I lived in. I was sure he could help me lose the pain, and get back to living.

I scheduled an appointment with him for October 12, 2009. Doctor AK, tested me with pain thresholds and watched me walk. I did what he asked me to do. I had to keep asking him to stop because I was feeling so nauseous. He would kindly wait until I said I was okay to do the next part of his testing. He confirmed that I had CRPS, and explained it to me, my mom, and my husband. He said there is no cure but there are some treatments. There is a chance of remission if caught early enough.

The first treatment we tried was nerve blocks. We did three rounds of nerve blocks. I felt the heat go down to my foot. He said that means it got where it was supposed to go. Unfortunately, after three rounds of nerve blocks there was no change.

By this time, it is 2010, and we started doing Ketamine treatments. I started with a three-day Ketamine treatment. Doctor AK, starts out low and slow. The goal of the three- days was to get to as close to 200 mgs as possible. It helped for a while. Then of course it came back. Four days at a time seemed to help more than three-days because of the low dose, and not being able to get to a high enough dose of 200 mgs. Because the insurance company said that Ketamine was an experimental treatment, they would not cover the treatment. I had to cover the expense myself. Luckily, I had some money saved and family helped out with the cost too.

I was one of the lucky ones with Ketamine. I did not get that nauseous. I did not really have any side effects besides being hot and being light sensitive. I had some dreams but he said that was "normal" and not to be upset by them. That made sense to me because he had given me Versed which made me sleepy, plus they always said sweet dreams.

Then came the end of the school year, and my principal called me into her office. She suggested I take a year off with medical leave because I was no longer able to be an effective teacher. I had been an exceptional teacher with her for three years. I thought to myself that makes sense. Maybe if I take a year off this will give my body the break it needs to heal.

The problem was that year changed nothing. Yes, the Ketamine helped with the pain but that was temporary. I was starting to have issues with quick temperature changes and passing out. I passed out in the shower, but luckily my husband was showering with me in our large shower for my safety. He barely caught me in time to stop me from hitting the tile hard. I still ended up with two black eyes, and the right side of my face was swollen. The CRPS went there next.

As my first year off of teaching was ending, I realized I was still in no shape to teach the next year. I had to sign up for one more year of medical leave. I knew I would lose my place at my school, which I loved, but I could still go back to teaching after this next year was up. I just did not know what school I would end up with. Little did I realize how wrong I was in that thinking. I was in complete denial of my condition of CRPS, and how much it was already affecting my life.

The second year of medical leave was ending and I had to talk with my principal. I had to stop teaching which really bothered me. I had to retire for medical reasons from teaching. At this point I lost my identity. I was no longer a teacher. I was unable to do much of anything for myself. I was just surviving. I was living for my son, and my husband, but not really for myself. I went to a pretty dark place like most of us do when we're told there is basically no hope of this getting better.

I had to apply for disability, because there was no way I was able to work. I had no idea how to do this so I just searched for a disability attorney to deal with all the paperwork for me. I interviewed one and was impressed with how well he knew the process. He explained it very well to me. He was very honest, and said that I would most likely be declined the first time. Most people are declined the first time, to weed out those who do not really qualify or want to deal with the hassle of getting disability.

At this point I was seeing a different neurologist who had been recommended to me. He was somewhat familiar with CRPS. He did a few nerve blocks trying to alleviate the pain in my back. The one strange thing about him was that no one was allowed to go back with me to talk to him. He said that took too much time. He was giving me pain medication to help with the CRPS, but that was not really helping. I was also on Lyrica and that was not helping much either. He was thinking I was dealing with carpel tunnel syndrome, but I had a Ketamine infusion, and the wrist pain that I was dealing with completely stopped. It was just CRPS pain, and swelling. He was totally surprised by that. Then he died in a car crash, and I was left with no doctor, and no way to get my notes from him for months.

My disability was declined, but they did note that they needed to have all of my records to be able to make a determination for or against me receiving disability. Once I finally, heard about where my records were and I was able to get them, we sent copies to disability for a determination. I was finally approved once they had all of the records.

Since I had lost my doctor, my primary suggested a pain management doctor. So, I started seeing a pain management doctor. He did know about CRPS. He did not believe in Ketamine, and I could either be treated by him or have Ketamine. I could not do both. I did not have the money to do both so I continued to see him. This was at the start of the Opioid crisis. My medications were counted. I had to have random drug tests to prove I was not a drug addict and taking illicit drugs. I never understood why he would think I would ruin my treatment plan by taking street drugs. One time I had left some pain pills in my weekly medicine holder and had to bring them back to prove to him that I still had them. I was shocked, and pissed! Of course, I did exactly what he wanted, and brought the container with me every time after that.

In 2015, I decided living in fear was no way to live! I decided one day to just stop living in fear and just do things anyway. If I was going to have to live in pain I might as well live to the best of my abilities. If everything was always going to hurt, no matter what I did, I might as well start living a life without fear of everything hurting me more because how could I hurt much more than I already was. Fear was controlling me and I wanted some control back over my life again. I started by walking on the sand at the beach while on vacation. I learned to pace myself and choose to do one thing each day.

In 2016, my husband and I decided to move to a house with a pool for therapy for me. I had been using a pool at a gym, but I found out the hard way why my doctor said not to go in water colder than 87 degrees. I put my feet into the pool, and it was not heated. The heater had broken but there was no sign about it. That is when the CRPS spread to the bottom of both feet.

While we were deciding where to move, my mom suggested that she move in with us to help us out with the house and help her at the same time. This was a great decision in so many ways. It helped my husband not to have to do everything around the house including cooking and cleaning. Mom was able to take the chores off of his shoulders. She was also able to help take care of me daily. She took me to appointments, so my husband did not have to take off work when I was unable to drive myself there.

CRPS affects both the person who has it, and the people around them, especially the family. They have to watch us be in pain, and not be able to do anything to help us. Back then I did not have the voice to say to my husband, "All I want is for you to just sit with me. I know there is nothing you can physically do to help, but just you sitting with me is more than enough." I know now that my mom taking care of me is her way of showing me how much she cares about me.

I was and am lucky enough to have family and friends who believed me, and who were willing to learn about what CRPS is. So many people are not that lucky. Having an invisible illness means many people do not believe you because they cannot see it with their own eyes. For most people, CRPS has never been heard of. It is as hard for them to imagine how a life full of that much pain could be real without being able to see it. It is hard enough to try and believe it ourselves, and we live through it every day.

My husband heard a commercial on the radio about a doctor in Clearwater, Florida who was doing Ketamine treatments, and who was also a pain management doctor. I was not impressed with the idea of a doctor who was advertising on the radio. As time went on my CRPS continued to spread and I was hurting so badly, I decided to look up the doctor my husband was talking about. My husband kept bringing up this doctor to help me. This doctor was Doctor AH. He actually would take insurance and treated patients specifically with RSD/CRPS and of course other pain issues also. The bonus was he was able to get insurance to pay for treatments. I scheduled an appointment to meet with him. I was impressed with how he listened to me and took the time to really understand what I was going through at that time. He knew a lot about CRPS. He was able to treat me and set up a treatment plan designed specifically for me. He explained the protocol he followed for a high dose Ketamine treatment. The protocol was over two weeks. The 1st week we started at the dose I had ended with from my prior treatment with Doctor AK, and increased from there each day. I had the weekend off from Ketamine infusions, but continued with Ketamine lozenges/troches on the weekend. The second week I was at the dose that worked for me all week. I slept really well after each treatment. He prescribed medicine to help me stay calm and for nausea. With his protocol I still did not have many issues with nausea. Once we added the patch behind my ear for nausea and a bit of dizziness, I did much better. I did have a headache afterward, but it was gone by the morning just like before.

In 2018, nine years after getting CRPS, my son told me about Facebook. I was like, "Why do I need that?" He said there were groups on Facebook, and maybe I could find a support group on Facebook. That made me think a bit, and I decided to give it a go. I had nothing left to lose at that point, so I searched for RSD/CRPS.

By this point I was considered full body. I had CRPS in both feet, legs, hands, arms, and part of my face. It was in this group that I found my voice and my purpose to live again. I found a community of people that I felt

154

instantly connected with on a completely different level. They understood me like no one else could. We had an instant connection due to having the same disease. I felt like, for once in my life, I belonged somewhere. I could make a difference in someone's life just because I cared enough to check on them. To respond to their posts and say I understand. That was a powerful moment for me! No longer was I lost in a sea of pain alone. I had found my tribe of people.

I was receiving Ketamine treatments about every two to three months at this point. After about a year of treatments it was getting even harder to start an IV in me. Eventually, to be able to continue to receive Ketamine treatments, I had to have a port put in. Getting a port was the best thing I had done to make life easier. Only one stick, not multiple failed sticks that just caused more bruising and pain.

I had a home health nurse come to the house at this point because I was not capable of getting around or driving on my own. My family and I both realized that I was no longer capable mentally of being able to drive. My brain was no longer functioning appropriately anymore. I was struggling with language issues and other cognitive issues. I was having migraines more often, almost daily at this point. Looking back, I am not sure if the light sensitivity and head pain was RSD or constant migraines. I was using a walker to get around because I had such bad vertigo anytime I turned my head there was a good chance I was going to lose my balance and have to catch myself. The world would go topsy turvy and I would lose my balance. My CRPS had spread full body including my head, face, the covering of my eyes, my ears, and even my throat. What I did not realize then was even my stomach, intestines, and lungs were completely numb.

At some point in 2019, a friend I knew from Facebook, who also had CRPS, told me about how she got into remission just by changing her diet, losing 80 pounds, and dealing with oxidative stress. At first, I was very skeptical and did not totally believe her. I thought, if it was that simple why didn't the doctors know this. I followed her on Facebook and called her every once in a while, for more information. I talked to her on the phone a few times over the next year.

Then during a particularly bad flare where I was in my room in the dark, with blackout curtains covering the windows, and still wearing sunglasses in the dark, no tv on and no music at all I found peace. I still cannot exactly explain how it happened, but I was able to be quiet and still during that time. I had lots of time to talk to God over the years about what was happening to me. I had come to the realization that at least I could help other people who were hurting and be there for them. In that ridiculous amount of pain, I realized that I did not have to react to the pain. I could just be in the pain, yet distance myself from the pain.

Then in August of 2019, came strangest pain in my head. It felt different from a migraine. It felt like it was inside my head. I talked to a friend, and fellow CRPS Warrior who used to be a nurse. She told me it was time to go to the emergency room(ER). That something was not right, and I should go to the ER. My husband took me to the ER. By the time we got there the pain was so bad, he had to push me on my walker into the ER. My head was killing me, and I had wrapped my arms around my head. They got me in right away. The nurse, and doctors were worried about a brain bleed. I got sent for a CT Scan. By the time I got back to the room I was in tears. The pain was just too much. I sat there crying for hours it seemed. I think I cried all the tears that I had not used since getting CRPS. My husband said the nurses would come and go, having to leave due to me crying so much and actually upsetting the nurses. They felt so badly about not being able to do anything until the results came in from the test. The results came back negative for a brain bleed. I heard the doctors say, "It's got to be a migraine. Let's give her the migraine cocktail." That's the last thing I remember. They also gave me medication to put me to sleep for a bit. The next thing I knew, someone was asking me how I was feeling. I was still thinking how did I end up lying down? The last thing I remember I was sitting up. I answered I feel better. They discharged me and sent me home.

The strange thing was that I was not feeling any CRPS pain at all anywhere! I told my husband but he did not believe me at all. It took three days for my family to believe me. I started walking around without my walker as much. I kept waiting for the other shoe to drop and for all the pain to come back. I actually cancelled my Ketamine Infusion for November. The pain stayed away for months before starting to come back at all. It started back in my head first and the buzzing came back in my feet and legs. I was back to being dizzy and dealing with vertigo again.

In April of 2020, I finally got the courage to ask my husband if I could try the program to lose the weight. It was the start of the food shortage in Florida, more than anything, that made me worry about having any food, let alone healthy food, I could eat with all my food allergies. It gave me the perfect reason to start taking care of myself, and lose weight in the process. I told him how healthy this was, and that my friend went into remission, and has been in remission for three years. He asked me to promise him I would stick with it. I actually said to him, "No, this time I am promising myself that I will stick with this." I was tired of being sick and tired, and very overweight.

In that moment everything changed for me! I finally started to put myself first. I followed the program exactly like they said to. In just five days I felt so much better! I finally started to have some energy! I was cleansing my body, feeding it healthy meal replacement shakes and learning to heal my body. I started to learn a lot more about how to eat healthy. I completely changed my diet. With the help of a holistic nutritionist, I began to eat a plant-based diet, and to learn what foods do not agree with my body. I started being able to walk again without being dizzy. Then I set a goal to walk around our small block. I was able to walk around the block with my husband holding my hand. Each new goal I set was a little bigger walking goal. First round the block, then the larger block, then half a mile and then a mile.

Now I walk a 5-K before breakfast six days a week. I have lost 80 pounds in 14-months, and a total of 110 pounds from my heaviest weight to now. I have not weighed 116 pounds in over 28-years. I go to the gym three days a week. I do yoga on Saturdays. I meditate daily to stay balanced, and calm. I am learning about ways to heal the body naturally. Changing my diet and learning to take care of myself first have been the two most important changes I have made in my life.

I learned about oxidative stress which is the underlying cause of aging and over 300 illnesses. There are over 20 studies done in PubMed about oxidative stress and CRPS. I found products that help with oxidative stress that have changed my life even more than losing the weight has. I have feelings in my body that I have never been able to express before. I never had the words for how I felt. Now I am learning even more about my body and myself.

I started, and have almost completed, a course in Strategic Life Coaching. I am going to use that along with my Master's degree in Varying Exceptionalities in special education to help children with disabilities and their parents through coaching, tutoring, social skills and support groups. My next course to take will be in executive functioning so I can really impact the children's lives more by being able to help them complete tasks, switch tasks, help with goal setting and much more.

For the next person diagnosed with CRPS, and for those still fighting with CRPS, do everything you can for your health. Eat as healthy as possible. Start eating gluten-free, no dairy, no sugar and nothing processed. Treat your body like a temple. Do everything you can to stay moving. Do not give up the fight for your health. Listen to your body. Pace yourself. You are not alone! We are all over the world! We are up in the sky in the stars. We are online. All you have to do is reach out. You are never alone.

P.S. Since being in remission I have sprained the same ankle again, and very recently injured my shoulder with no recurrence of any CRPS symptoms.

A FALL INTO A BUNKER LEADS TO CRPS

Tina Ortiz

My complex regional pain syndrome (CRPS) story began in the middle of the desert on the border of Iraq. It was the first night of the war back in 2003, and the alarms were going off regularly alerting us to possible incoming bombs, and chemical weapons. We were in and out of the bunkers in full gear that included our gas masks, helmets, and Kevlar all night. During one of the visits to the bunkers, the sand gave way under my right foot causing me to move in a forward motion while my left foot, and leg remained behind me. This event caused the labrum in my left hip to tear along with some cartilage. The subsequent pain in my hip and groin continued throughout my stay in Iraq and when I returned home.

It was the ongoing pain that brought me to the Orthopedist at Portsmouth Naval Hospital in Virginia. After several tests, including an MRI where dye was injected into my hip, I was diagnosed with labral tears requiring surgery. A hip arthroscopy was done in November of 2004. Soon after surgery, I began to have numbness and tingling in my toes, and lower leg. The Orthopedist at first thought I was overdoing it during physical therapy (PT), so he reduced my number of visits. Despite the change in my treatment plan, one evening I experienced severe pain, and my left leg turned bright red. This pain felt like flames and electric jolts at the same time. I could not wear any clothes and could barely place a sheet on my leg. Simple pain medicine would not relieve the pain. When I spoke to the Orthopedist the next day, he told me he suspected I had reflex sympathetic dystrophy (RSD) now known as CRPS. He prescribed Neurontin and referred me to a Pain Management Specialist at Bethesda Naval Hospital (now Walter Reed National Military Medical Center). It was there my diagnosis was confirmed.

My long journey with CRPS has taken me to many different specialists and through many different treatment plans. I have been prescribed Neurontin, Lyrica, Celebrex, Tramadol, and Topamax. I have also had Epidural Injections and three failed Spinal Cord Stimulator (SCS) trials. Finding the right medication combination took time. I am now on Lyrica, Celebrex, and Topamax, which keeps my symptoms moderately controlled for the most part. The trial, and error of my treatment plan did not come without periods of immense pain, numbness, tingling, "bee stings", "electric jolts", and swelling. It also resulted in the progression of my CRPS to my other leg, and lower back.

Today it has been almost 17-years since I was first diagnosed with CRPS. I continue to live with daily symptoms and regular flare-ups. The flare-ups consist of intense pain, redness, burning, "electric jolts", and the inability to place anything on my legs even a thin sheet. I try to avoid flare-ups by taking my medicine, and by avoiding stress, prolonged activity, and cold temperatures. I used to take Tramadol during the flare-ups, but it is no longer prescribed in part due to the Opioid Crisis. Fortunately, medical marijuana is prescribed in my state and the topical cream, and tincture helps lessen some of the pain.

Because my CRPS had progressed, causing me tremendous pain, and limitations with my ambulation (losing my balance and difficulty walking due to pain, swelling, and numbness, also an inability to do our physical fitness tests), I decided to retire from the military after 22-years. I truly loved the military and the job I was performing as a Commanding Officer and Nurse Practitioner. This was a painful loss for me that I still feel today. Now I am teaching nursing students virtually. Although, CRPS tries hard to steal everything from you, I refuse to let it steal my love of nursing, and sharing it with the next generation.

CRPS is part of my daily life now. I often find myself waiting for a flare or for it to progress. Simple procedures such as dental work often result in more pain than what the average person has. I recently had a dental implant done, it actually was my second one, the first one went great with no complications, but this one was full of pain, swelling, adjustments, and now a constant ache, that the dentist chalks up to my quenching and having TMJ. But with my history of CRPS, I cannot help but wonder if my CRPS has decided to move into my jaw. It is exhausting sometimes because you do not know whether to just accept it is CRPS, TMJ, or do you go back to the dentist, or doctor because you know something is not right. It is also exhausting when you ask for help, and do not get it. A few years back I was having a lot of flare ups and asked my PCM for a pain management referral. She told me no, that my medicine could be adjusted by her first. So, she made some dose changes to the same medications that I had been on since 2008. These changes only provided a temporary relief. So, I asked my Veterans Affairs (VA) doctor about a year later when I had read about the use of Ketamine, and other treatment options by the VA. He agreed to submit a request to the Veteran's Medical Center Pain Clinic for which he also received a no. The recommendations they provided him with were all ones that I had already tried. At this point, I was so frustrated and disappointed. I feel as though I am left to stay on my current treatment plan without the possibility of benefitting from any potential advances in the care of CRPS patients. I also worry about the long-term effects of my medications on my body. I counter this worrying by keeping myself informed, eating right, reducing stress, and exercising when I can.

Support groups help so much. Talking to people that know what you are going through, and can empathize means so much. Although, my CRPS occurred from an injury that is different than many others, I know I am not alone in this fight. Whether, I participate in person, or on social media it helps to share my struggles, or to commiserate with another people. I also feel good when I can answer another person's question, or help them in some small way. CRPS is a heavy weight, but it does not have to be held up by one person. We can help each other. I am thankful for that.

MY JOURNEY WITH CRPS
Kelly Kane

I have enjoyed helping others for as long as I can remember. Becoming a nurse was an easy career choice for me as it combined my love of helping with a strong fascination with the human body and how incredibly resilient it is. I graduated from nursing school in 2009, passed my registered nurse (RN) boards the next month, and landed my first RN job in February of 2010. I have always been an overachiever so it should not have been a surprise that I went straight to work on a Neuro Intensive Care Unit. I immediately noticed two things about working in the ICU: First, I was absolutely fascinated with the critically ill patients we had, and loved learning about the complexity of each case. However, with those severely ill patients came a heavy load of stress, and unpredictability that made me feel sick to my stomach every shift. In addition to the high levels of stress, the physical demands of the job were taxing in every way. Lifting, turning and caring for patients who are in a coma and on the ventilator left my body aching and tired. I got into a routine of soaking in an epsom salt bath as soon as I got home from work. When that failed to give me relief, I started taking ibuprofen with my meals. Then I split up my shifts, so I would have a day or two off between working, to give my body a rest. My lower back began to hurt all of the time. I dreaded having a heavy patient on the ventilator because I knew my body would pay for it afterwards. Then one night something changed. I was at work, and was miserable with back pain. After repositioning my patient, I went to sit down in my chair to do some charting. I immediately felt tingling down my left leg along with intense pain. I could not sit down on my chair. My charge nurse sent me home that night. Little did I know that would be my last night working as an RN.

My primary care doctor gave me NSAIDS, Vicodin, and Flexeril muscle relaxers. Nothing touched the pain. I was miserable. It took two weeks to get an MRI, which showed that I had torn a disc at the L5-S1 level. I was unable to do much for myself living alone. I made the difficult decision to give my resignation at work, and relocate to Oregon to be closer to my parents while my back healed. I would get a job in Portland after my back was better. My friends helped pack up my apartment, and scheduled a moving truck to transport my belongings from Arizona to Oregon. I had a lumbar steroid injection to help me get through the excruciating two-day car trip up the coast to Oregon. After arriving at my parents' house my pain started to change; my left leg was still tingling but also felt heavy. It is hard to explain but almost like my limb did not belong to my body. My back was extremely sensitive to any kind of touch. I could not handle someone walking up behind me without bracing myself. I started putting ice packs on my back at night, so I could sleep. Finally, someone suggested that I try acupuncture. I was hesitant at first, but I was willing to try anything to help lower my pain. I did not feel any relief from acupuncture. After my seventh session, I got up from the chair and felt "off." My mom was waiting in the car for me since I was unable to drive myself.

The pain and sensations that I felt on that car ride home are something I will never forget. I felt as if every nerve fiber in my body was exposed, and raw. Any bump in the road, no matter how big or small, made my pain level spike so high that I could not speak. I was tingling all over, and wasn't sure if I was having a stroke. My Mom wanted to take me to the emergency room (ER). Instead, I asked her to pull the car over. I slowed my breathing down, and told her to just get me home. I carefully climbed into bed, and knew something was not right with my body. What I had just experienced was terrifying. A couple of weeks after the acupuncture appointment, my partner suggested we drive to the coast. I had never seen the Oregon Coast, and they thought it would be a good distraction. The coast is about 90-minutes from my parents' house. We set up pillows, and blankets so I could lay down in the backseat. This became my new way of car travel. The scenery did not disappoint! I walked around for about 10-minutes, and then my pain spiked. I quickly noticed a burning sensation in my left foot. By the time we got home my foot felt as if it was on fire! I could not believe what I saw when I took off my socks and shoes; a bright, cherry red foot that was literally hot to the touch. I did not understand why my foot was red and looked sunburnt?

I took a picture of my feet because it was so odd looking. The next day while taking a shower I looked down at my feet. I yelled for my mom to come into the bathroom. My left foot was mottled looking bluish, and purple with strange red spots. Now what is wrong with my foot? My RN brain started trying to figure out what could be the cause. I had seen mottled feet on my patients before. They either had a clot in their leg, or the patient was in the process of dying- neither of which are good scenarios. I went to urgent care to get checked for a blood clot which was negative. My primary care doctor gave me a referral to see Doctor G, one of the best neurosurgeons in the area, for a further assessment. I thought I would get some answers for sure with this appointment. Unfortunately, that could not have been further from the truth. After explaining everything that had happened with my back injury, pain, and strange color changes of my left foot, Doctor G, condescendingly looked at me and asked, "So, you said you are a neuro nurse?" I nodded my head yes. He continued, "Then you know that color changes in a foot, or limb have zero to do with neuro, right?" My heart sank. I walked out of there not only in high pain, but with low confidence in the medical system that I had once been so proudly a part of. I sat down and googled my symptoms to see what could be the cause. Something called reflex sympathetic dystrophy (RSD)/complex regional pain syndrome (CRPS) came up, but I did not give it much thought because it looked horrendous, and I had never injured my left foot.

DIAGNOSIS

My primary care doctor suggested I see a neurologist named Doctor S. My appointment with her was on February 15, 2012. My mom drove me, and waited in the car. Doctor S, was easy to talk to, and we immediately clicked on how we geeked out on the brain, and how fascinating it is.

After a thorough assessment, she did two tests on me: a nerve conduction study and an EMG (electromyography). Both were within normal limits. Towards the end of my appointment, I showed her the picture of my bright red foot after my trip to the coast. I described the burning feeling, and also how my foot looked mottled while standing in the shower. She looked at me and said, "Have you heard of CRPS?" I told her that it had come up on a google search, but I had ruled that out because it looked terrifying and my foot was not injured. She said, "Kelly, you have many of the classic CRPS symptoms. Some people develop CRPS in different ways than others. This looks like CRPS. And, if it looks like a duck, and walks like a duck, it probably is a duck." I walked out of that appointment feeling numb. My Mom asked me what was wrong when I got into the car. I could barely get the words out. When we got home my stepdad was waiting for us to hear about the appointment. I burst into tears and collapsed in his arms sobbing uncontrollably. I felt helpless and terrified. I stayed in my room for the next couple of weeks with the lights off, and drapes closed. I screamed out to God asking, "why me, why am I being punished?" I cried until I could not cry any more. Darkness had taken over my world and I had never felt so scared. How was this happening to me at the age of 34? I finally reached out to one of my dear friends to tell her about my diagnosis. While we were on the phone, she found the RSDSA (Reflex Sympathetic Dystrophy Syndrome Association) page on Facebook. She encouraged me to reach out to them for support. I remember feeling sick inside as I nervously wrote a post on the RSDSA's page: "Hi, my name is Kelly, and I was just diagnosed with CRPS. I do not know much about it, but I am very scared, and I feel alone." Within an hour I had several people who had replied to my post. The first person wrote, "Hi Kelly. My name is J. I have had RSD for 17-years. I will be your friend, and help you any way I can." I burst into tears. It felt surreal that there were others like me who understood what this pain felt like. Little did I know that J, would end up not only being my advocate, and cheerleader, but also one of my best friends.

TREATMENT AND MEDICATIONS

My new friend J, told me to get into a pain specialist ASAP, to get a sympathetic block. She also shared her experience on which medications had helped her in the beginning of CRPS. She emphasized to me the importance of accepting that I will always be in pain, even after taking my medications. That was a hard lesson to learn. Two months after my diagnosis, I received my first sympathetic nerve block. I had incredible results! They attached thermometers to my feet before, during, and after the sympathetic block. After the procedure was over my left foot, which had previously been burning hot, had dropped more than two degrees Celsius. I was over the moon with happiness! While this first block only reduced my pain for three months, it allowed me to start physical therapy (PT) and learn how to use my left foot again. Working on desensitization with my physical therapist was crucial for my recovery. When I started PT, I could only wear fuzzy socks, and my Croc shoes. After a couple of months of desensitization, I was able to wear a pair of athletic shoes for short periods of time.

Unfortunately, during the next six months the CRPS climbed up to my left calf, and also spread to my right foot. I also developed allodynia on my left arm. My pain doctor in Portland, Doctor S, prescribed many medications for me such as anticonvulsants, opioids, lidocaine patches, compound cream, muscle relaxers, etc. I had two more sympathetic blocks during my first year of CRPS, until they no longer were effective. I have had PT on and off throughout my years with this disease, and have tried countless promising medications and alternative healing practices. My mental health suffered greatly each time a new symptom would appear. Anxiety and fear would take me spiraling down into dark places. I had lost my nursing career, pride, and felt like a shell of my former self.

HOPE AND HEALING

Four years after my diagnosis, I began working with a physical therapist who had 25+ years of experience with CRPS patients. She had me work on a Graded Motor Imagery (GMI) program. I thought it was a bogus technique that was probably wasting my time, but decided to give it a try.

During this time, I also started to challenge myself to walk more, even if it increased my pain and put me in bed for the day. I began with walking a half block to the park in my neighborhood. That led to being able to walk one lap around the park. I hated every step as I felt the flames on my feet. I will never forget the day I made two complete laps around the park. I immediately sat down on a park bench, and took off my socks and shoes, a common practice when I knew my feet were blistering from the CRPS. I was in so much pain, but also beaming with pride at my progress. It was during this time that my marriage ended, which was earth shattering at the time but ended up being a blessing in disguise. I was free from the heavy stress, and unpredictability of the relationship, but felt like damaged goods with a chronic disease. My pain skyrocketed. Bone pain, muscle spasms, allodynia, and sleep deprivation had set in and it had me in a fetal position. My mom packed up my belongings, and took me back to live with her, and my step-father.

The next chapter of my life was like a reset button. I started to make significant changes that I believe are partly responsible for how I am doing today. I stopped putting any alcohol, or substances into my body and began to make healthier food choices. I went gluten-free and dairy free. I admittedly was skeptical of these diet changes, but had read they might help with inflammation. I sat less, moved more, and got busy. The changes were gradual. I was in high pain and had to take breaks throughout the day, but noticed that I needed less medication and had fewer high pain days. I found myself in a healthy, loving relationship with someone who accepted me, CRPS and all.

As my mental, and emotional health improved, so did my physical abilities. My progress over the last five years has waxed and waned. I still have flare ups that will land me in bed. But today I do not live in 24/7 pain like I once did. And, today I do not take nearly the amount, of medications I used to. I am in the process of renewing my RN license, so I can get back to my career of helping others, something I never thought was possible after CRPS. I wish I could go back nine years ago and tell my scared, newly diagnosed self to have hope that life can get better. But perhaps I would not have been able to hear that. A few lessons I have learned on my journey thus far; to take my health one day at a time, find gratitude in the littlest of things, and to not let my diagnosis become my identity.

"THIS GIRL IS ON FIRE"
Catherine Pento

It was a beautiful June morning in 1999. I was having my coffee putting on my nurse mates, scrubs etc., getting ready for work. Oh, how I loved working with the elderly, and the disabled. I was working for the visiting nurse association. I went to the office grabbed my daily paperwork, and assignments, then I headed out the door on my route to my first stop. My first patient was doing great and having a good day. Everything was fine. I checked the patients BP, and checked for bruises in case of any falls etc.

I got to my second patient; she was trying to ambulate from her bed to her chair by herself. Unfortunately, she started to fall. When she was falling, she grabbed me by head, and neck area. That is when I heard something pop. I said to myself oh, this is not good. I went back to the office, and had to do an accident report. My supervisor decided to send me down to the local walk-in clinic they said, oh it must be a sprained neck, and they gave me muscle relaxers (valium) set me along my way. Months later I was still in severe pain I went and saw a specialist Doctor H, well unfortunately, he found out that I had several issues going on. I had four ruptured disc. He stated this is not looking good. Doctor H, handed me paperwork about CRPS he said not only do you have all these issues, you also have radiculopathy, and needed another ganglionectomy after the surgeries I just had. He wrote in my chart I was quite handicapped, and needed many surgeries. He fought with the insurance company for about a year. Finally, they agreed to let me have the surgeries, however by then it was too late. I had no use of my right arm, and hand. I wore a neck brace for three years. The saddest day was when Doctor H, stated there was nothing more

172

that he could do for me, my nursing career was over. I felt like my life was over.

It is now 2000, I went back and forth to pain clinic, after pain clinic. I tried Tens units, nerve root blocks, special creams made with lidocaine. They could not do a dorsal spinal stimulator because of my allergies to metals. Every medicine you can think of I was on. As most of us have been on these horrible medications (I am sure you know what I am talking about). Not a good time at all. My body hated the side effects of these medications. Now I needed medications to stop me from being sick to my stomach. It is a never-ending cycle.

Let's move ahead a few years, it is now 2009. I was taking care of my mother at the time, she had a cancerous head and neck tumor, and unfortunately, she only had short time to live, and you got it, I was the primary caregiver. OMG, how am I going to do all this by myself? My husband worked 70-hours a week. I reached out to the VNA, and I got the help I so needed. At that time, I was not able to dress myself, let alone take care of someone else (my mom).

I was putting clothe soap in the refrigerator, and doing odd stuff. I could not type, could not speak properly, and I am thinking it was all the stress of my mom, and I being sick. I chalked it up to just being that. Meanwhile my siblings decided to do the most un-thinkable to their sister who is apparently" nuts" they wrote the Medical Board saying I was being over medicated, and given to many narcotics. No one knew at that time I had a BRAIN TUMOR. (Family can really kick you when you are down). We hired six lawyers from Boston, and had my doctor's name cleared of any wrong doing. She was also my mother's doctor. Pretty sickening ha? LET'S JUST

173

PUSH OUR SISTER RIGHT OVER THE EDGE. Unfortunately, my mom passed away in July.

At the end of August 2009, the same year my husband was putting in a window, and I was at the hospital because I lost my eyesight, while driving my vehicle. They thought I was having a stroke. Come to find out I had a brain tumor. I cried could not believe I had a brain tumor. Then within two weeks it grew to my brainstem, and my nasal cavity. It was almost inoperable, but they resurrected the brain tumor (a success), so I thought.

A year later my head still would not close up properly, and heal the way it should. The doctor then decided after I told them I was allergic to metal. That all the metal and the screws would have to be taken out now. My daughter was getting married, and I was to walk her down the aisle (that story is for another day or book). The doctors agreed to allow me to be at the wedding, however that Monday following the wedding, I was back in for my second brain surgery.

I was in a Boston hospital lying in bed, and my husband had called me. I was screaming my bed is on fire, my bed is on fire. Well at that point they(all the doctors had all agreed that my CRPS had gone full body. So, I did not know what to do? I was ready to put up a quarter of a million dollars to put myself into a three-day coma in Connecticut, with the hopes that it would help settle my pain down. My pain level on the score of one to 10 was always a 10. My husband did not like the idea that I was going to go into a coma, I may not come out of, at the tune of $250,000 (it's only money) what is my life worth? My best friend I will call her Sissarooni. She and I decided we would research everything, and anything about CRPS, we printed out so much paperwork, anything and everything we could find on this ugly beast. I was very lucky I had a great doctor. Doctor S, decided to listen to us with all our research papers printed up on a funky lime green polka-dotted envelope. Lol! We really caught his attention. Well, I started a three-day Ketamine infusion. I had lots of ketamine, and so many other medicines that could kill a horse. I was doing these treatments every three weeks. I went through these Anesthesia pain specialist treatments for about 9 to 10 years, they helped. They did not cure me, but took the edge off, and got my pain level down to around a six. Then this doctor, and the team of all my specialists decided that the best thing for me would be to move out of cold weather. I lived in the Boston area, and the winters there can be brutal. It also affects the CRPS. Oh, I love my Boston. I love my doctor's but the cold does not like CRPS, fibromyalgia, and the other issues I have. Taking a shower is like having rubber bullets on me. A ceiling fan feels like it is cutting my skin open. The doctors also stated I be in a wheelchair by the age of 60, if I did not get to a warmer climate.

In 2016, my husband, and I decided that it was time for me to no longer continue to suffer any longer. We relocate to Florida, we moved here five years ago, and it has helped. We researched, and found qualified doctors to help. I was pleasantly surprised how many doctors down here were aware of CRPS. Not every day is perfect, but so much better. Unfortunately, with this move came with a lot of animosity from my family. They just could not understand how I could possibly get up relocate, and leave my grandkids and family. What other choice did I have? Did they even care? Some friends may have thought it, but never said anything. What would you do if it was you? I did what I felt was right for me. We had plans on retiring here in our later years anyway. If anyone that has this horrific condition, please do what is best for you. Follow your instincts be your own advocate, and make sure your doctors hear "YOUR VOICE" ! No one ever wants to live with this condition. I could go on and on, I will not as we all know our stories are pretty much the same

175

especially, when it comes to excruciating pain. So, the next time someone decides to tell you it is all in your head, ask them if they would like to live the lifestyle that you have to live. It is not called the suicide disease for no reason .

I have spent a lot of days being in bed, not being able to go not being able to attend a wedding, or an event even concert at times. On the good days I try to really enjoy my life to its fullest. Some day's it is a living hell. I was just told three months ago that my CRPS is now in my right foot. Yay said no one ever.

But I will never give up! As much as this ugly condition rears its ugly head, I fight back or at least give it my all. It is not my nature to quit. At least I can research from a bed or home. I send you all gentle hugs, and prayers that someday they will find a cure for all of us, and the ones who will have to hear these horrible four letters-CRPS.

MY ELEVEN YEAR BATTLE WITH THE
MOST PAINFUL CONDITION KNOWN TO SCIENCE

Jasmine Marie Miller

On May 2, 2010, I was at summer softball practice with my team. I thought it was just another normal day... Little did I know that this would be the day that would change my life forever. I was covering second base, and I went to catch the ball, my glove fell off, the ball hit my left wrist. It was instantly on fire, purple, and swollen. I knew something was not right. My dad came to picked me up, and he took me to the walk-in clinic. They took x-rays, which showed it was not broken, and they put a brace on it, and referred me to an orthopedic specialist.

On May 6, 2010, I went to see Doctor B, and he looked at my wrist he said I had something called complex regional pain syndrome (CRPS), also known as reflex sympathetic dystrophy (RSD). He wrote it on a sticky note, and told my mom to go home and look it up on the internet. We did and it was horrifying. I was only 13-years-old, and I did not know what most of those words meant. I did not understand why I was in extreme pain, and why I was not improving? My left arm was stuck in the same position for a year. I could not move my arm, or wrist at all. No one could touch my hand, even the slightest breeze would bring me to my knees in agony.

I was referred to a pain specialist in Columbia, MO in fall of 2010. Doctor M, wanted to try a stellate ganglion nerve block. The block did help take my pain away for five days. When those five days passed by my pain returned with vengeance. They did another block, this time it did nothing.

177

I was then referred to physical therapy(PT) to work on strengthening my hand and to lower my pain levels. I had many sessions of PT, and still I was not progressing like I should have been. The pain began to get worse. It travel up my arm, down my neck and into my back. It progressively worsened until February 2012. I woke up one morning and could not walk, nor move my left leg. At that point I was on fire throughout my whole body. I was put into a wheelchair while we went from doctor to doctor in Missouri trying to get answers, but as usual they do not understand CRPS. My mom thought it would be in my best interest to not wait around, and she drove me to the Mayo Clinic emergency room (ER) in Rochester, MN. I was then admitted to the services of the Mayo Clinic. I had appointments with many specialists, and underwent two weeks of intense physical therapy where I had relearned how to walk again. Because of the hypersensitivity, they thought that it would help to desensitize my nerves by rubbing different fabrics, and sensations on my skin. That was pure torture, and did not help at all.

In March 2012, I started the three-week Pediatric Pain Rehab Program (PPRC) at the Mayo Clinic. It was a program for teens with chronic health issues that kept them from being able to live a "normal" life. My mom and I went through the program together. All of the parents would have classes on how to parent teens with chronic health issues. They would tell our parents to discipline us if we talked about our pain, missed school, or work, unless we were bleeding or had a protruding bone, then we should not miss anything. Now I do not agree with this but I am very thankful for the friends I made at PPRC. Though it did not help my pain, it did help my outlook on life (not to focus my life around the pain).

I returned home in April 2012. At that point, my pain was still out of control, and I was referred to another pain management doctor, who only recommendations were to either try a spinal cord stimulator(SCS), or to go to either Mexico or Germany, to try the ketamine-induced coma. We did not like these risks so we kept searching for other safer treatment options. My mom stumbled upon Calmare Therapy; a type of biophysical "scrambler" technology that uses electrodes placed on the painful areas to try to re-program the brain to receive a "no pain" signal instead of a "pain" signal.

In the Fall of 2012, my mom and I traveled to West Warwick, RI to receive treatment. At, this time I was diagnosed with CRPS in all four extremities, and at this point it was now affecting my eyes. I was diagnosed with bursitis in both of my hips, carpal tunnel in both wrists, and tendinitis in both knees. The multiple sessions of Calmare Therapy, which did help for a short period of time, and it reduced my pain from an eight to a ten, and it gave me back my ability to function, and I was able to graduate high school in my junior year in the spring of 2013. With many treatments over time the nerves find new pathways, and what has previously helped has now stopped working.

In February 2014, I had heard about a doctor at the Carolina Pain Institute, who had experience in treating CRPS. At my first appointment seeing Doctor N, I was given only two options, either have the ketamine infusions or the SCS. So, I decided to go ahead, and try the SCS trial. It helped tremendously.

In June 2014, I had a four-lead spinal cord stimulator implant. I had finally had some relief with the SCS, my daily pain was down to a three out of a

10, on a normal day. I felt I could handle more on my plate. I went to work, and enrolled in college courses. A year later my pain flared back up, and my stimulator stopped giving me relief, and began causing many other issues. In 2017, I went to my local dentist, and he was unable get my mouth numb enough to fill a few cavities because of my CRPS. The dentist decided to refer me to an oral surgeon who ended up removing five permanent teeth that could have easily been fixed. My SCS began to shock me, and shut off randomly, as my pain areas were no longer getting coverage. The representative for the company who makes the SCS came in, and hook my battery up to a tablet, and diagnose the issue. I was told that it was impossible for the stimulator to shock me.

After many issues, pain, and five surgeries, I decided to have it removed in October 2019. At this time, I was able to leave the physically abusive relationship I had been in for the last two years. My pain was now uncontrollable. I could not get out of bed, and one morning I woke up and could not keep food down anymore. I went to a G.I. specialist in Missouri, and had many tests done. Unfortunately, all the results came back normal as they always do with this condition. I was told there is nothing else they can do for me. From November 2019 to June 2021, I could not keep anything down not even water. I would pass out randomly, my vision would go black at random times, and I hardly left my house. I was miserable to say the least. After seeing over 30 specialists begging for help, and being told they just do not know what to do. I lost over 120 pounds very quickly with no answers. I was giving up hope.

In March of 2021, I found a Neurosurgeon who kept pushing the PRIALT pain pump implant. I went through the process to be approved for surgery, and had the trial done before the permeant implant could be placed. On

April 16, 2021, four days before the implant, my dog bit me. I waited about four hours before going to the hospital. I woke up, and my right hand was throbbing, swollen, and it did not look good. I decided to go to the ER. Within an hour being there I was told I had a torn tendon, and I had six different infections, because of my weak immune system. I was rushed to emergency surgery, so I would not lose my hand. I spent four long days admitted to the hospital. I still was not eating, or drinking. I was starving to death, my body was shutting down, and I was down to 105 pounds. I begged for a feeding tube, but because anything going into my stomach causes extreme pain, and nausea. None of the doctors thought it would be in my best interest to do it. After four days I begged my healthcare team to discharge me to go home. I was in a really dark place with no hope, and no answers. The only thing that has kept me sane, and gives me any relief from the pain is medical cannabis. I have tried many different treatments over the years from many prescription medications, physical therapy, procedures, implants in my spine, changing my diet, exercising, acupuncture, essential oils, and counseling, but I have found that cannabis is what helps the most even if it is a band aid for the pain. I am not going to sit around and suffer.

On June 1, 2021, my mom and my boyfriend decided I could not wait, as I was down to 105 pounds, the light was fading from my eyes, and my body was giving up. I no longer had control of my bladder. I was weak, and in extreme amounts of pain from head to toe. I was taken to the Cleveland Clinic to get some answers, but I still did not get the help that I so deeply needed. I was told the same thing as the other places, that it's a type of physiological illness that has been proven by science many years ago not to be true. I was told to go to counseling, do biofeedback, and do physical therapy. I was told if I follow this plan, I would have remission in two years.

Well, six months later, I had very little improvement, and my doctor wanted to send me to a pain rehab program.

Since June, I have been back home. I have gained 10 pounds, pushed myself to get better, which has flared my CRPS up. I am back to eating every couple of days due to my stomach pain and nausea. The pain is unbearable, and I am not able to sleep.

On October 19, 2021, I flew to New York for treatment with Doctor Glenn Gittelson, hoping I would finally receive the answers I have been searching years for. I had been asking many doctors to do an MRI due to neck, and head pain. I was told it was unnecessary. When I arrived to New York, my pain was unbearable from traveling. On my first visit with Doctor Gittelson, he performed a peripheral nerve block, and within twenty-minutes my CRPS pain from my head to my toes was now gone along with all the symptoms I had. My vision came back, and I could see perfectly, my cold and pale body now had color and warmth again. My muscles were relaxed. I was overjoyed I had ZERO pain. I had never been able to say that I had zero pain before over the past 11-years.

On Friday October 22, 2021, I had an MRI of my cervical spine and my jaw. Doctor Gittelson sits in the room with the technician, and reads them himself. Doctor Gittelson sat down, and explained the results of the MRI with me in great detail, and he answered all of my questions. I have found no other doctor that has done what Doctor Gittelson does. Doctor Gittelson goes after the mechanical triggers, and what is keeping your sympathetic nerves lit up, and addresses those triggers, then the peripheral nerve blocks shut down the sympathetic nerves. The MRI confirmed that my cervical spine at the C-1 level is out and rotated from past domestic abuse I suffered from.

On October 26,2021, my C-1 disc was put back into place. The MRI also showed that I have severe temporomandibular joint (TMJ) damage on both right and left side of my jaw. Science proves that my jaw stopped growing around the age of eight years old from trauma. The last few days my pain has flared up pretty bad because of the weather, and getting my C-1 put back into place. Today Doctor Gittelson gave me a broader peripheral sympathetic nerve block. As he explained it to me, rather than blocking individual peripheral sympathetic nerves, he blocked the superficial cervical plexus, known as an Erb's point block. The relief I received was more profound than the other blocks. I was pain free for five hours! I had no pain from my head to toes. I was no longer cold and pale, but I had warmth and color again, I have never felt the way I felt today after this nerve block. It was very strange not being on fire, and in agony for once in the many years of suffering with this condition.

The next day I flew back to Missouri, and I will return in a week for more treatment. One of the reasons CRPS patients have these bad flairs that do not go away, is because they are usually caused by a trigger that keeps the sympathetic nervous system active in a dysfunctional manner. These problems can be either physical, mechanical or biochemical. In my individual case due to trauma, I have a significant cervical spine issue that we began treating non-surgically, and due to trauma, I have an injury to my jaw joints that does require surgical correction. I have to have a bilateral discectomy with a fat graft replacement to fix my TMJ. My bones are deteriorating, and is cutting off the blood supply. These two injuries

183

that I sustained, as Doctor Gittelson explained to me is what has kept my CRPS symptoms in such a high active flair for many years. The nerve blocks I received, and the relief I got from them are an indicator of the more sustained relief I should get once these two mechanical injuries I have are corrected. I know now that there is an objective scientific way to diagnose, and treat CRPS patients. As Doctor Gittelson, told me at my first appointment all pain can be traced to a source. I finally received my answers and received some relief! I am finally getting the care I so desperately needed years ago. GOD IS SO GOOD and he answers prayers, you just have to hang on to hope. There is light at the end of the tunnel for me it took 11-years.

Many do not understand CRPS, and the horrible pain that overtakes our bodies, and how it can be the most painful condition known to science, but we look "normal" most of the time. Unfortunately, families and relationships start to fall apart because they cannot understand why you are not getting better after years of battling this disease, and all the doctor's appointments and all the bills. Having a severe health condition especially, CRPS is extremely isolating, and others make you feel like being with you is inconvenient because they miss out on fun things, because they have to take care of you. In the end they end up having enough, and giving up which only leads to more stress, pain, guilt, and grief. It is a horrible spiral. CRPS is nicknamed the suicide disease, after many years of suffering, many patients take their own life. It breaks my heart that along with the never-ending pain, many friends, family, and loved ones do not believe that it could be this bad. But they just cannot understand because they have not experienced it.

My whole outlook on life has changed, the small things where what mattered the most. On this journey I have lost so much, and have had every right to give up years ago, but I held on tight to the thinnest strand of HOPE that I had. Knowing that my prayers would one day be answered. I hope by telling my story, it would help at least one person to know there is HOPE, if you just hold on.

Luke 1:78-79 Because of the tender mercy of our God, by which the rising sun will come to us from heaven to shine on those living in darkness and in the shadow of death, to guide our feet into the path of peace.

I dedicate my recovery to my beautiful friend Jenna.

USING MY VOICE TO RECEIVE THE TREATMENT I NEEDED AND TO SPREAD AWARNESS FOR COMPLEX REGIONAL PAIN SYNDROME (CRPS)

Melissa A. Adams

Hi, my name is Melissa Adams. I live in South Carolina with my husband, Thomas, and our five pups. I am a complex regional pain syndrome (CRPS) warrior, cancer survivor and gastroparesis fighter!

But today I am telling you my complex regional pain syndrome (CRPS) story.

I started having problems with my left foot in 2014. It started as just pain; it then grew to where I could not walk on it. So, I was referred to an orthopedic doctor in February 2015. I was sent to physical therapy. I did this for six weeks. Unfortunately, I was getting worse instead of better. I was walking with crutches, and started to have to end activities that I truly enjoyed. Not being able to walk on my own, and the pain was also affecting my work. So, my orthopedic doctor decided that the next step would be surgery.

On May 5, 2015, after over a year of foot pain, I had my first Achilles surgery. On this day, my husband drove me to the hospital, we were sent to our room. We met with the doctor, and I went in for the surgery.

After the surgery I was sent home, bed rest for two weeks. After two weeks I went back to see the doctor, to have the cast taken off, and get fitted for my boot. This day was a terrible day. It plays in my mind over and over still to this day. I needed to go to the restroom, and wanted to try to help myself. Even though I was not supposed to. I got to my destination and got up and went to wash my hands. A scream that my husband and daughter had heard me throughout the house. A scream that is so indescribable. They got me in the truck as quickly as possible. My husband drove me to the emergency room (ER). Every movement, every breath was excruciating. The staff at the ER got me right in. I was given a shot of morphine. The ER did not have an MRI, so I received an X-ray. The doctor could not see anything that caused any concern. My pins were where they were supposed to be, and nothing else showed up. I was sent home for bed rest until I was able to see my orthopedic doctor. I had my appointment with my doctor on Monday. The event occurred on Saturday. I was still in so much pain, and I knew that it was different. The x-rays were looked at in the ER, and I was given some more pain pills, and sent on my way. I shortly got into a deep depression. Because I did not know what was going on, and the PAIN! The pain was so terrible. I could not explain it. It was days of crying and screaming. It was the hardest two plus years for all of us.

I kept complaining to my husband, daughter, and doctor about my pain. How different I felt. I would bring this up at every follow up appointment. But all I would hear was that I am healing, and the surgery went well. I was soon sent to physical therapy. My physical therapist is amazing. They all are. They worked with me and went at my pace. Which was not fast enough for me, but I was doing what I could. I also let them know about my pain. How different I felt. How I was falling, and I was not able to put pressure on my foot. Even after all these weeks, months of "healing". My PTs kept telling me to stress this to my doctor. Which I have. My PT emailed my doctor, and expressed the importance of seeing me. Also, for an MRI to be set up. My orthopedic let me come in for an emergency

187

appointment. He was not happy with me. He gave me another X-ray, and said all that he could see is density in my left foot. Well, hello I could not use my foot! He told me to keep up with PT and to take it easy. I was healing, the surgery went great. I was still complaining and the pain, swelling, and discoloration was so severe. My PT even wrote an email to my orthopedic about his findings. But still, I am healing. Finally, after a year of complaining, because of my doctor wanting to wait a year so I can "heal". I received an MRI. The MRI showed that I had tears in my "new" Achilles, and hair fractures in the heal of my foot.

With this finding I was told by my orthopedic to keep wearing my boot. Nothing changed! I am still fighting, and trying to find my voice so someone would listen. The outcome was another surgery. In September 2016, I received what I hoped was the answer. It was not! I was in agony! PT was again starting, and oh the pain! Pain was not even the right word. But I pushed myself. I finally took my first steps; agony is not the word, but I do not think they make a word that is right for CRPS pain. I was so proud of myself though. I could only take a few steps, and it is still the same to this day. This time around with PT, I had an AMAZING PT who was fresh from college, and held on to my every word. She worked with me and tried every "trick" she knew. Trying to get me to the point of being independent, and able to walk and be out of the terrible pain that I was in.

As she worked with me, she also noticed the swelling, and discoloration. She asked me if I noticed it, I told her yes. Then she asked me if my doctor noticed the swelling and discoloration. I again told her yes, and that he tells me it is part of my healing, and that that both surgeries went great. She looked at me and asked if I ever heard of complex regional pain syndrome (CRPS)? I told her no, but this was not the last time that I will hear these words. My PT then asked me to make an appointment with my orthopedic doctor. She wrote me a note to give to him, and told me she was going to email him too.

I made the appointment, and was able to get in the same week. When I got there, the doctor let me know that he received the email, and I handed him the note. He told me that he does not believe that I have reflex sympathetic dystrophy (RSD). Then he explained CRPS is a new term for RSD. If I want the medical field to listen, I should use the term RSD. I am healing, and this pain is all in my head. I needed to push myself more. I had enough of him telling me this, that I am not in pain. I am fine! I am healing! I just could not take his sarcasm anymore. I asked him if he could please refer me to someone who could help me with this. He did. He wanted to just get rid of me. I was referred to a pain specialist. But, my orthopedic doctor, sent me for a nuclear imaging scan first. So, I had another appointment with my orthopedic and he again said he does not see where I have CRPS. But he has reached out to the pain specialist. I just have to call to make an appointment.

I called to make an appointment as soon as I left the office. An appointment was set, and I had hope in my heart. It was two weeks later, April 2017, and I was there with my specialist. Who confirms that yes, I do have complex regional pain syndrome (CRPS), I was finally diagnosed with something, even though I was scared about CRPS, because I did not know anything about it, I never even heard of it until now! Yet, I was relieved at the same time. I was so happy to have someone that listened to me, and I have been diagnosed.

I started treatment by doing ketamine infusions. We also started with different medications. Still to this day we are trying to find what will help me. I have done so many trials. From continuing PT, water therapy, deep dry needling, Acupuncture, more medications, and different types of injections. I even stayed in the hospital for 10-days on a Ketamine drip. It feels like every time someone gives me advice, or a suggestion to try something, my response is, "Yes, I have done that."

I am still with the same pain specialist. He is so nice and listens. It is too bad I do not deal with him at my appointments. I must deal with his nurse practitioner (NP). She does not listen, like my doctor does. It is the same thing over and over with her. Do not get me wrong, she is a nice person. But as a NP she is not the best. Unfortunately, she talks about the same thing as if it is new. She tries to mix up my medications, like it is new. She forgets to put in my prescriptions, and always tries to put the blame on someone else. There is so much I could say. But I would run out of room. But I use my voice with her. I stand up on things that she just puts aside. By using my voice and standing up, I saved my life a few times. But that is another story.

I am going in for another injection, to see how it does. The last three I had almost a year ago did nothing! But I am crossing my fingers.

I am also looking for a new doctor that can take me on. Unfortunately, so far, I cannot find someone who prescribes Ketamine. I need that prescription to help keep that edge off. It helps with the burning pain. That burn inside you that you cannot control.

Because of the medications, dry mouth and severe reflux, I now have problems with my teeth. I have broken a molar in half and my front teeth just keep chipping. I also have had my first cavities. At 40-odd-years old. I just got eight filled. This is all because of side effects from CRPS, and of course medications.

I have now lived with full body CRPS for almost four years now, and my left foot is going seven years. From my feet to the top of my head. I swell, turn red, black, and blue. I burn all through my body and have not had a dream for almost seven years now. Due to not being able to sleep. I only can take a few steps until my foot shoots a pain throughout my body that I cannot describe.

I survive every day, by speaking my story, spreading awareness, and listening to other CRPS Warriors. I do this on groups that I have found on social media, and I have also started my own Podcast. "CR(a)PS: A Day In The Life Of A Woman With CRPS." If you ever want to reach out, and do an episode, Look me up! ☺

As a CRPS Warrior, I know the pain, the loneliness, the exhaustion. But I also know the support, and love of family and friends. The community that we have for each other. The strength I find in myself. I am thankful every day for this. Trust me, some days are easier than others. There are those days that I just cry, so I cry, and it is okay. I just ask you to remember that after that good cry, remember to reach out. Because you are never alone.

I also just want to shout out to all those that stayed by my side, and kept me going. Lifting my spirits and myself up! To my husband, kids, family, friends, and caregivers. Thank you! Thank you for all you do. Plus, thank you to me. For listening to my body, and for using my voice!

LIVING WITH COMPLEX REGIONAL PAIN SYNDROME TYPE II (CRPS-II)
TWELVE YEARS WITH THE DISEASE THAT KEEPS ON GIVING
Christina J. Dowds

My complex regional pain syndrome (CRPS) started in August of 2009. In June 2005, I was injured whilst performing duty as a police officer in Northern Ireland. My police vehicle came under attack from a group of youths who threw bricks at us. I was hit directly on the left side of my face with one of these bricks. Further to this I was the victim of yet another assault whilst I was carrying out an arrest, in February 2006. On this occasion I received a blow to the left side of my face, struck by the young male I was arresting. This resulted in me suffering a dislocated jaw. Thankfully my jaw relocated by itself, and did not require hospitalization - on this occasion, but did leave me in a great deal pain and discomfort.

After a few months of this pain and discomfort, my General Practitioner(GP) referred me to a lovely maxillofacial surgeon. This gentleman suggested that a bite guard was required to help me heal. I found this a bit uncomfortable to wear at night, but I persevered with the bite guard, hoping it would resolve my pain. Unfortunately, for me when I went back to see the doctor, I discovered he was retiring. To continue my treatment, he referred me to another maxillofacial surgeon. I was also pregnant at this time with my youngest son. I could not go through any further treatment, or tests for the period of my pregnancy.

In October 2007, my beautiful son was born. This allowed me to continue with the treatment for my jaw injuries. I made contact with the new surgeon, who sent me for an MRI and CT scan. On receipt of the results of these scans, I was informed that my injury was so severe that I required surgery to repair my jaw. In June 2008, I agreed to this surgery. Let's face it I am not medically qualified so I went on the advice of this surgeon. The first surgery was to 'flush debris' out of my jaw joint. This surgery did nothing for the discomfort I was in. With this first surgery not being successful, I was informed that I required a further surgery. I underwent this second surgery in August 2008. This surgery was much more intrusive. I had my left jaw opened up from the top of my ear to the bottom. The surgeon did explain to me that my left eye could droop after the surgery, but this can correct itself. When I woke from the surgery my face had dropped on the left side but came back after a few days. Unfortunately, now, when I am extremely tired, swollen and sore, my left eye will droop again. This can be very embarrassing, as it is very plain for people to see, and it is something which I cannot hide. No amount of make-up is going to cover that up! Again, this surgery was of no help, in fact I was left in even more pain.

In August of 2009, I was told I needed a further surgery. I was initially informed that this operation would be a 'bone shave' to my jaw. However, while waiting to be brought to theatre (operating room), the surgeon came to speak with me and my husband. He asked me did I know what I was going to be done, I said yes, 'I am getting my bone shaved'. At this, the allegedly very 'eminent' and 'highly respected' surgeon became very confused, and described a totally different surgery which I had never heard of. When I became upset, he told me "that would be worst case scenario." He then left the room in a fluster, and I was taken down to the operating theatre

193

When I came around, I discovered that 'worst case scenario' had become a reality. I had a reverse question mark opened on the side of my head and down my ear again. He had opened me up in my hair line, so I only knew he had done it when I touched the side of my head. During this operation he had removed my meniscus, this is the shock absorber in your jaw joint, and allegedly grafted my jaw muscle over the joint. However, it became abundantly clear to me that this had not worked, and the surgeon returned to examine me, he informed me that this surgery had yet again not been successful. I now required a procedure to fully replace my jaw on the left side. He further informed me that he was not able to perform this surgery and I would have to travel to England to have the surgery carried out. As you can imagine I was devastated with this news. To be honest, at this time I was not prepared for any more surgery, and had begun to seriously doubt the medical profession.

After my surgery I continued to consult with this local surgeon, The pain in my jaw and face was now unbearable. My face was burning, the pain and was visible as my face was red and swollen. He told me he did not know what was causing this, but still began to prescribe a plethora of different nerve pain medication.

Finally, in 2011, he referred me to a pain management specialist. At the first consultation I was diagnosed with complex regional pain syndrome-type II (CRPS II). This pain specialist went through a list of certain medications he wanted to prescribe to me. When I told him that I had already been prescribed these medications, he was very shocked. I was already being treated for CRPS by my surgeon who was telling me he did not know what it was!

I went back to my surgeon and asked him some very uncomfortable questions which he really did not want to answer regarding my treatment and care. I stopped seeing this surgeon at this point.

Unfortunately, in 2013 I was involved in a serious road traffic collision. As a result of this collision, I suffered a fractured sternum and seven fractured ribs. Unbelievably, these injuries were not initially diagnosed by the treating hospital, and I carried on my working life as well as caring for my son, not realizing I was so badly injured. I attended my own GP because I was in so much pain, but they kept telling me that I had had only suffered muscle damage. All this with having my face totally on fire, and in agony all the time.

In 2014, I eventually decided that I had no option but to undergo the jaw replacement procedure. I really did not want to do this, as I had been treated so poorly by the previous surgeon and the medical profession in general. However, I could not have been so wrong in my worries. The new surgeon in England was fantastic! He guided my husband and I through every part of the surgery, and I felt very reassured moving forward.

All this time I had still been performing my day-to-day duties as a Traffic Police Officer. I cannot tell you, how much I loved my career. I felt a thrill each time I pulled on my uniform and stepped out into that police vehicle, not knowing what each duty would bring.

However, once I decided to have my surgery, I was moved to a desk job, as I could not take the risk of any further injury. I was devastated - to say the least!!

I travelled to England in April 2016, to have this jaw replacement surgery. The worst part of this was having to leave my children at home in Ireland. My two older children, who were in their teens, understood but still worried about what I was going through and how I would look after getting this operation. My youngest son who was only nine at the time was very upset at me having to leave him. Before I left, I had to put a lot of planning into the time I would be away from my children, I had to organize childcare, meals, and the day-to-day running of the house. It was like a military operation.

I was terrified and very upset, even though I was totally informed of the procedure I was still concerned as every operation has its own risks.

Arriving at the hospital, I was made to feel so welcome and treated extremely well. I cannot fault the staff or the surgeon at all. After the surgery the surgeon explained to me that I had osteoarthritis in my jaw because the previous surgeon had caused so much damage to my jaw joint. My husband and I had our suspicions regarding my last surgery, but his information confirmed the concerns we had regarding my previous care and treatment.

I was supposed to stay in hospital for over a week post-surgery care. However, I was back home in Ireland with my children four days later. The surgeon and anesthetist were both surprised at how quickly I had firstly, come around after the operation, and secondly how quickly I was recovering. Even though I was treated so well I just wanted to get home to my children and my own surroundings to heal. I was devastated at the scarring on my face which went right under the left side of my jaw line to the center of my chin. The surgeon had prepared me for this but I think nothing prepares anyone for anything until they see it. I looked like Frankenstein's bride!

My hospital room became a meeting point for all the nurses after they found out that I was an injured police officer from Northern Ireland. I cannot explain how this act of kindness made me feel during this difficult time. Many of the staff were also injured veterans, both police and military. One of them was even a battlefield medic who was retraining as a nurse! Their comradeship and understanding was so helpful to me.

Unfortunately, the CRPS continued to get worse. The jaw replacement procedure had caused more trauma to my facial nervous system, even though the surgeon had been so careful. I still travel to England for treatment, and to visit my surgeon, who keeps a careful watch on the condition of my prosthetic jaw joint. I have to be so careful not to get any type of infection as it could live on the prosthetic joint. I have to visit my dentist regularly which is very painful as I only have limited mouth opening now.

I have since discovered that the initial injury to my jaw was not as severe as the surgeon who began surgery, had said. I should have been treated simply with a bite guard and counselling. I have now been left for the rest of my life in excruciating pain. I do not trust the medical profession at all and question everything I am told. This actually overflows in the care of my children as well, if I have to take them for any kind of medical treatment, I will question the doctors. I have also been medically retired from the Police Service. I loved my job so much, and I feel I lost everything I had worked so hard to achieve. This has been the most painful part of this whole process to lose my job which I had wanted for so long.

I sometimes feel so worthless, that I am not providing for my children by doing the job I loved. My youngest son was only 11-years old at the time I was medically retired. This disease has taken so much from me, and left me with so much pain and anger. I am bad tempered with everyone, and can snap at the smallest of things. I know I am doing it and still cannot help it when my pain is a 10 or above.

After being prescribed morphine for pain relief, which I was not taking anyway, I decided to search for more natural holistic ways to help me with my pain. I have discovered medical cannabis, which does help. I am now involved in lobby groups trying to get the UK government to prescribe this medication to sufferers of chronic pain conditions. I also exercise very regularly, even though it hurts so much to do. My children and my wonderful husband, who have been through this journey with me, are my strength. I am now trying to find a new kind of normal for myself and my family one day at a time.

CRPS VS. MY LIFE AS A MEDICAL ASSISTANT
Brenda Needham

My life as a complex regional pain syndrome (CRPS) patient all began in June 1999. I had applied for life insurance; all the paperwork was completed. The only thing left to be done was the home physical. I also had to have blood work done. They called me to schedule a date to have this all done.

The technician came to my home. The first test was to record my height, weight, blood pressure, pulse, and respiration for the blood work.

The technician tried six times, yes you heard me six times, and no blood. I normally do not allow someone to attempt to draw my blood this many times but my thoughts were if she got no blood then I would not get any life insurance.

So, on the sixth blood attempt in my right arm, there was instant pain right away. The needle had hit the medial aspect of my arm into the veins, causing a voltage shock going up into my arm. I yelled for her to pull the needle out right away which she did. She did not get any blood from me that day, she advised me to put my head between my knees, and take some deep slow breaths.

She told me she would send into the lab what she had, which was just my height, weight and urine test, but no blood work. She also mentioned to me that she would have her supervisor call me for further appointments to finish up the insurance physical.

As the night went on, every time I would extend my right arm, it was just like a voltage shock once again over and over and over. It was becoming where I was constantly rubbing around my middle finger and/or squeezing my finger to make it feel better. This lasted for about four days.

I was then at work at the hospital, working as a medical assistant, and it was bothering me to the point, I rubbed it so much, I developed an open raw sore on my finger. I went and spoke to my Faculty physician, and he asked me what had happened? I explained my situation what had happened with the blood draw, and the voltage shock in my arm. He knew right away what had happened. She hit a major nerve in the medial nerve in my right arm. He called up to the pain clinic, and spoke to the anesthesiologist, and I had an appointment that afternoon for my first nerve block, which had confirmed my diagnosed of having complex regional pain syndrome (CRPS). This was in November 1999.

What does a nerve block mean? The stellate ganglion is part of the sympathetic nervous system that is located in your neck or either side of your voice box. A Stellate ganglion nerve block is an injection of medication into these nerves that can help relieve pain in the neck, head, upper arm, and to upper chest. How is a nerve block done in the neck? During a cervical block the doctor injects a pain-relieving medication into the nerves in the neck. It is usually a combination of a local anesthetic and cortisone used in the injection. The anesthetic numbs the pain, and the cortisone reduces the swelling.

How long does a nerve block last for a CRPS patient? Nevertheless, nerve blocks are used for their ability to produce long lasting pain relief to those with mild to moderate conditions although every patient is different, generally speaking. Nerve blocks for chronic pain management can last anywhere from anywhere from not at all, to six months, or up to a year. Are nerve blocks painful?

All patients are given IV catheters within sedation medication to help relax, and then numb the skin prior to the nerve block placement.

My first nerve block, I must not have been completely out because, afterwards for two weeks my throat was sore. When I went in for my second nerve block, my anesthesiologist told the nurse to give her more sedation to knock me completely out, because I kept swallowing. Anyway, I had a total of nine nerve blocks in my day.

Then my symptoms of CRPS were spreading to my left side of my arm. My physician sent me to have an EMG which is an electromyography nerve conduction velocity study. This was to rule out carpel tunnel syndrome (CTS). After this test, I went in to speak with my physician, and he informed me that I did not have CTS, but I must consider CRPS. I wanted to pass out. Yes, my worst nightmare it was spreading. I was sent to the Mayo Clinic in Rochester, Minnesota to be part of a study there, that dealt with a medication study treatment for people with CRPS.

They were doing a study at Rochester Medical Center for people who had CRPS in multiple limbs, so that fit my description. A cancer patient that was taking a medication which I cannot remember the name of that drug, but it was helping her CRPS at that time she had CRPS, she was still diagnosed with cancer as well.

So, they wanted more research to the study. Fifty percent of the people had that drug, and fifty percent did not. At the end of the study, I found out that I did not have the drug, and I found out that my CRPS was spreading to my legs. I went back to Mercy Medical Center in Cedar Rapids, Iowa, and had more nerve blocks done in my lower half of my body.

At this time, I was walking with a walker, because my legs were not strong enough to hold me up. My doctors were talking about doing a spinal cord stimulator (SCS), but before I could have this SCS implanted, I had to go through studies before having the permeant one placed. This meant having a trial SCS temporarily implanted. I spoke with the surgeon, the neurologist, and with the anesthesiologist for going ahead with this procedure, and I had to talk to my insurance company before, we went ahead with this procedure.

I had three different trials of the SCS implanted. Before I had my SCS trial placement done, I had to do a lot of physical therapy, occupational therapy, learning to walk ,learning to open and close my hands. Touching each finger to my thumbs that was a struggle due to the skin tightening, and sensation of my skin being a painful feeling as though you sometimes felt as though you had no skin on your flesh, and as if someone was rubbing a piece of sandpaper into your wound.

One of my therapies which I had to do was to put ice-cold water on one side of the sink with ice cubes in it as much as I could tolerate, and on the other side of the sink ,I had to put in hot water as much as I could tolerate. Then I had to place my entire hand, and arm in the one side that was very cold and leave it in as long as I could tolerate it. When I could not tolerate it any longer, I would submerge my arm and hand into the warm water, and keep in there as long as I could. I would keep going back-and-forth with the cold and hot water to help desensitize my skin. My other type of therapy was taking different types of material, and having to rub it on my skin to help desensitize my skin as well.

One of the other types of therapy I would do was to get some type of rubbery type of substance that Occupational therapy would have. Some of them would be harder than others, some of them would be not so hard depending on the color of the rubbery substance. Some of the therapists would hide different types of objects in the putty, then they would have you tried to find the objects with your fingers. This would help stretch my fingers during therapy.

Due to the CRPS, my skin became very painful to touch. I could not tolerate having anyone hug me, because it would cause me more pain. When I am in the grocery store picking up cold refrigerated items, it would feel like the coldness was burning my skin. In the winter time I had to wear multiple socks because my skin would be very cold.

I am now on my second SCS, my first one was a Medtronic stimulator, which only had one lead, which means that it was only for my right arm, and that is the only thing that it would help control the pain. I had this implanted on May 20, 2000.

That SCS lasted until May 20, 2014. At, that time I had a new model implanted. It was made by Boston Scientific. This model was a four-lead model which would control my upper arms, both of my legs, my back, my chest, and my neck area.

I had lost many jobs during this time of having CRPS. I worked as a medical assistant in the hospital for many years. I graduated from Kirkwood Community College in 1989, as a medical assistant. When I was first diagnosed with CRPS in 2000, I had to leave my job due to all the pain, and treatments that I had to endured.

My life now, is good. My CRPS is in remission, but I still struggle with having the thoughts of my CRPS coming back.

At, times I still get pains in both arms, but it is mild. I use my stimulator often, and I still go to the paint clinic.

I always do research to further my knowledge about CRPS.

So, thank you for allowing me to tell my story. I hope that this will help others

MY CRPS STORY
Veronica Warren

My complex regional pain syndrome (CRPS) story started on August 31, 2018, when I was lifting and carrying very large, and heavy cartons. One of the cartons was wide in girth, and very heavy, so I had to stretch my arms as far as I could to accommodate the box.

I felt the strain, but it did not hurt until the next day. It started in the middle of my forearm, and gradually spread from there to my hand, so that I could not use my arm, or hand for anything. My primary care physician (PCP) gave me a prescription for a narcotic pain reliever. The pain continued for weeks, and my PCP had me see an orthopedist.

He diagnosed me with carpal tunnel, and he did surgery for it. He also gave me gabapentin, which was useless for the intensity of pain I was experiencing.

Next stop was to see an arm, and hand specialist who told me the problem was further up my arm in the **pronator teres muscle (which is located on the underside of the forearm). This new doctor recommended I have surgery to repair this muscle.** So, I had my second surgery, which again did not relieve the pain.

My next stop was to see a spine and pain specialist, who sent me for several tests and procedures....none of which helped me.

My frustration level was high because I lived every day with the same pain. I was referred to the head pain doctor, who told me it could possibly be complex regional pain syndrome (CRPS).
I had never heard of CRPS before, and after he questioned me about my symptoms, he concluded that I did have CRPS.

I had three nerve blocks done, then later, I had three other different types of nerve blocks, which only helped me for a few hours.

So here I am, now three years later with the same pain, and symptoms as I started out with. I am currently on hydrocodone 10/325 three times a day.

This is a bad situation, since there is no cure, and my life is day after day of pain and misery.

Thank you for the opportunity to share my experience with CRPS.

UPDATED STORY SECTION

In this section of the book, we will include updated stories from patients who have previously submitted their story in past volumes in our CRPS Book Series.

These stories, are to update the readers of our past volumes on how the patient is doing, and what changes they have had in their life, since their original story was first published.

UPDATED STORY

"A WARRIOR'S SURVIVAL- SHANNON'S STORY...

SHANNON'S HOPE FOR HOUSE CALLS AND HOME MEDICAL CARE"
Shannon E. Killebrew

In September of 2019, I was humbled and thankful for my story to have been included in Volume I of this wonderful series of publications. It was an honor to share my 13-year journey as an CCRPS warrior at that time. CRPS has taken an enormous toll on my life and I truly hope sharing my experiences will help aid with the awareness we so desperately need in our battle with this disease. The medical community is lacking the proper knowledge and expertise to help many of us on our journey. My name is Shannon Freeman Killebrew, and this is the update of my survival story.

My story began as sudden horrid pain in my right knee, and progressed within six weeks to my requiring a wheelchair. Within one year, I had severe limitations with my arms and hands (from overuse of crutches endeavoring to stay ambulatory), dental and oral issues (leading to a severe restriction in diet and speaking) and a spreading of the CRPS. I became bed bound requiring 24- hour assistance in 2016.

At the time of the first Volume publication my story ended with the forming of my patient Advocacy for Statesboro, GA., U.S.A., and beyond. Shannon's Hope for House Calls and Home Medical Care was born, and was my passion. My advocacy was born from a vital need. My need. My need to have physician house calls, home medical care, and reliable caregiver assistance.

The founding of my advocacy occurred nearly a year after I was discharged from my long-time primary care provider after three decades as an established patient with his office. The reason cited - I failed appointments. Yes, I did, technically. I will now explain this in further detail.

The Story Behind Shannon's Hope

Like many CRPS warriors traveling had always been very difficult, the pain from the vibration of my car alone was horrible. I padded the floors, under my feet with pillows in an attempt to absorb some of the vibration. The movements required to get in and out of the vehicle were beyond painful. The person driving me had the arduous task of assisting me, handling my wheelchair, loading it, and lifting me (in my wheelchair) over thresholds, curbs etc. I had lost my ability to drive within the first weeks of the CRPS onset, there was absolutely no way I could tolerate the pain from using foot pedals. I will not even begin to discuss the emotional and psychological toll of losing my ability to be mobile independently, drive my own car and the stares of strangers because I was "that" person in a wheelchair. It was all too much! And, this was before the CRPS spread beyond my right leg and the systemic effects of the beast were everywhere.

Fast forward years later when my health has declined dramatically. Despite valiant attempts to adapt my life to my new reality, it has become impossible to travel. My body was too fragile. The vibration of a moving vehicle, the stress of being manipulated in and out was all too much. Not to mention one of my preexisting diagnoses was Solar Urticaria, a severe allergy to sunlight. I had always controlled it fairly well with medications and light therapies - until CRPS! After CRPS, apparently my immune system was too weakened. Sunlight was unbearable. I then began the decline to allergy of artificial light. This cemented my fate... Travel was of detriment, and impossible.

I knew I had to see my physician. I endeavored via numerous medical transport companies and non-emergency ambulance transports. I finally, found a wonderful non-emergency ambulance transport who felt they could accommodate my needs, with a signed release of all liability and an out-of-pocket fee of $1,774.00 (which was not in my budget) for the 12-mile round trip transport. They would not be able to merely drop me off and pick me up, they would need to stay with me. We tried. I was now unable to travel beyond my neighborhood entrance, with two paramedics, due to extreme symptoms. Paramedics deemed it unsafe. I was distraught.

I needed to see my physician. I needed my medications. One friend suggested the unthinkable, could I travel in a hearse on a stretcher? The ride may be smoother. After the initial shock of the idea wore off, local funeral homes were contacted. They were each very sympathetic, but denied the request for obvious reasons.

However, could you imagine the sight of arriving at your PCP's office in a hearse!! Yes, I was desperate.

I realized travel was no longer in my realm of possibility and another avenue must open. I knew I was likely not the only person who risked their already fragile health to try and see their physician for a five to ten minute "face to face" visit. Something has to change.

My mission is to use my experiences and struggles as a bed bound dependent CRPS warrior to pave a way for all who are homebound, bed bound and unable to travel without severe difficulty to have access to physician House Calls and Home Medical Care such as serology, imaging etc. Our community of warriors has such unique needs and awareness is crucial. CRPS is so misunderstood, misdiagnosed and under treated. There is a severe lack of knowledge in the medical community as a whole.

I never would have imagined 15-years-ago, when I first became unable to bear weight and walk, this would be my life. Today, I feel my purpose is to create a legacy and hope from my heartbreak, pain and losses. I lost every dream and aspect of a normal life to CRPS. Survival has been my goal for the past 15-years.

My dreams of being a Veterinarian were dashed. I changed my college major to my second interest and completed my BBA in Accounting (focus in forensic accounting), yet my career aspirations as a Forensic Accountant were also dashed. God had other plans.

The last two years have been an amazing experience! I had absolutely no idea how to begin this endeavor. I said a prayer, followed God's lead, and created an advocacy group with a blog on Facebook.

There have been very difficult aspects of this journey. I had long "hidden" my struggles, my health and my declining body from the world. I did so to avoid the ostracization, questions, labels, discrimination and misunderstanding that often accompanies health warriors when we speak of our needs. My energy was also quite limited and prioritization of my daily activities is pivotal. However, I soon discovered a vigor in advocating!

I loved creating posts that not only told of my struggles, but let others know they are not alone. I discovered graphic art applications on my little phone where I could design my own images and graphics. The one finger I type with was up for quite a challenge! I have quite severe limitations physically. To this day, I am still learning new techniques every day within these apps.

MY ADVOCACY GAVE ME A PURPOSE. IT GAVE THIS BED BOUND, TOTALLY DEPENDENT, PERSON, WHO FELT HOPELESS, A PURPOSE.

I have been honored to have met and connected with extraordinary warriors from not only my local community, but across the USA and now internationally! I never fathomed I would be so blessed in this endeavor. To know these brave, strong and courageous souls is a joy of riches. The miles melt away when I chat with someone who understands, truly understands. We are a support to one another.

So many are bed bound, home bound or have severe travel restrictions like myself. So many are in need of physician House Calls and Home Medical Care. In recent decades these were a staple of medical care. The medical community was devoted to the well-being of the patient. Physicians knew that traveling was very taxing on an ill or fragile person. Somehow, the humanity became lost as healthcare began a metamorphosis into a business with a goal-profit.

Pleas from myself, my family, social workers, legal aid services and caregivers did nothing to persuade my physician to perform a house call or offer telehealth. I was terrified. This was not medical care. This had morphed into discrimination of the disabled and those with health limitations.

THE STRESS OF SEEKING MEDICAL CARE SHOULD NOT EXCEED THE STRESS OF THE ILLNESS/DISABILITY/DISEASE.

212

It has been an arduous journey. I have used precious energy and my health has greatly declined as I pursued every lead for house calls, mobile serology etc. I am literally alive today, to type these words, as God worked through a dear friend who assisted me across state lines. Thousands of emails, calls and letters led to a physician willing to travel five hours round trip to my home! The concierge fee is quite exorbitant as you can imagine. My friends have been ever faithful to raise the funds for each appointment via fundraisers!

There are numerous benefits to the patients, physicians and insurance companies. Medicare especially is encouraging home-based care. The following benefits are documented by numerous sources:

- Pivotal germ control during the very hazardous cold and flu seasons.

- Limits exposure of fragile patients to contagious individuals in an office setting.

- Increases the quality and care the patient receives while in the comfort of their, accessible home.

- The physician/patient relationship is stronger.

- Significant reduction in Emergency Department visits due to routine care being maintained comfortably and efficiently for patients who would otherwise go without care and resort to the ED when health declines.

- Significant savings to insurance companies, hospitals and the patient as in-patient care costs are reduced. (Many are hospitalized due to health issue exacerbations which could have been managed by routine care).

- The patient is no longer required to go to a long-term facility in most cases and can remain with their family for greater longevity and quality for life.

- Physicians are allowed greater reimbursement vs. in office appointments reducing the need to limit their Medicare and Medicaid patient base.

- Specific ICD codes for insurance billing serve as an incentive for both patient and physician.

The Ongoing Process

It is still a process as my physical limitations are numerous. I have very little arm and hand use. I'm legally blind as the symptoms in my facial area won't allow me to wear my glasses. I cannot speak above a whisper without severe pain. Presently, I am trying to procure a mobile phlebotomist for routine blood work. I am now following up on a lead for a company who offers mobile imaging and serology in home. I am thrilled about this prospect! Over the last two years the accomplishments have been amazing. I am thankful for the following accomplishments:

- Correspondence with a concierge medical service in Savannah, GA., willing to serve my area (when covid is no longer a threat).

- Procured a mobile phlebotomist for areas near me.

- I have assisted people as far away as Seattle Washington, to have mobile blood work in their home.

- My advocacy had been featured on podcasts in Savannah, GA.

- Invited to speak at local City Council Meetings. (my statement was read on my behalf by a City Council Member and others with disabilities were there in support).

- Enjoyed the privilege of Shannon's Hope for House Calls and Home Medical Care to be listed on the International RSD Foundation website.

- Coordination with the American Pain and Disability Foundation (APDF) in their advocacy efforts.

The most unexpected blessings have also occurred. As, I endeavored to be a voice for everyone needing home based medical care, I found my voice in so many other areas. I had long hidden away from the world... hidden myself, my experiences and my traumas.

I never dreamed it would expand to be a safe haven for warriors. We are free to discuss our traumas, experiences, fears, hopes and ideas to help one another. So many have suffered grievous physical, emotional, mental or financial abuse (often all of the before mentioned) at the hands of their caregivers or providers.

So many suffer from PTSD, and have been conditioned to remain silent regarding their needs for fear of further ostracization, discrimination or labeling.

I am honored that so many brave warriors feel comfortable sharing their stories and triumphs in my patient advocacy group. Silence can be deadly. In breaking our silence, we are simultaneously creating a voice and raising the awareness needed for reform.

I have made it my mission to be a voice. As such I speak not only for myself, but for all others, even outside of the USA. I also focus on reform and better educational curriculum for caregivers, as many of us require them. The turnover is great within home health agencies and private pay as well. Continuity of care and stability is imperative to one's health. For most, this is not occurring and already fragile lives are under enormous stressors as a parade of strangers enter their homes in the name of care. Cancelations are way too common often leaving dependent persons without a means of nutrition, hygiene and daily needs.

We often feel as if circus animals on display. Guinea pigs of sorts as new people learn and train with us. We are in our homes, in our "safe place". Yet, we are forced to open our homes, our belongings and our bodies to strangers in the name of survival. We pray and take a chance... with each new person. I cannot describe the anxiety, and often PTSD, we face with each new hire that may or may not be a proper fit even after exhaustive training and exposing of our most private daily moments. With each new person and energy lost we decline further. We lose more of ourselves. We lose more of our spirit. Some opt to go without care versus the before mentioned.

Better educational curriculum is key for both the patient and the caregiver. A more disciplined and informational curriculum would better endow the future caregiver with the knowledge needed. Many are overwhelmed and ill prepared due to no fault of their own. This only adds to frustration on the caregiver's part and often results in less-than-optimal care to the patient.

The need for patient centered care is so great! People go without basic medical care daily as they cannot travel. I have corresponded with physicians in an attempt to understand the roadblocks which are prohibiting this care for so many. I have yet to receive any answers. I wonder if the issue is logistical, financial, legal or otherwise? All I do know is that people are being ostracized and this must stop. The people in the greatest need are being ignored essentially.

A recent study by the Students with Disabilities Advocacy Group (SDAG) at my local university, Georgia Southern University, found the number 1 request by disabled students in my community to be "treat me as a human". I will let those words sink in!! For people of such a young age group to have already been exposed to such ostracization and discrimination speaks volumes.

Treat me as a Human

A good friend of mine is the president of SDAG, a graduate student and media director for our Mayor. SDAG has asked if I would coordinate with them on increasing accessibility accommodations in our community. People should be able to access sidewalks, elevator buttons, public restroom doors, ect. I am thrilled for this synergy!

217

I have also been actively pursuing palliative care for myself and others. Palliative care is a separate discipline and not to be confused with hospice care. It is for those with life-long chronic illnesses and it provides clergy, psychological support, possible nurse oversight etc. It is meant to relieve the suffering and improve quality of life for people of any age and any stage of serious illness, whether curable, chronic or life threatening. Palliative care is meant to be an extra layer of medical care and can be used in coordination with one's PCP. Unfortunately, it is proving quite elusive for many CRPS warriors and others with chronic severe illness.

There is a phenomenally enormous gray area of vitally needed care between the healthy and the terminally ill. This gray area is leaving enormous numbers of people without routine or palliative medical care. There is also an issue of accessibility for those in non-urban areas, as well as those without affluent connections. To deny adequate pain relief and support networks is unconscionable.

I had recently initiated correspondence with a newly established local palliative care program, via a local hospice, in hopes of finding this care for myself, others and more information. After a rather impatient wait on my part, I was absolutely appalled at the reply I received. The reply was that "local physicians told her that the disease is complex beyond their expertise - so it would be improper for them to try to treat it. She said the best resource would be a peer-support group for the disease that she found on the internet. It's just one of those situations where the only resources are in major metropolitan areas with large medical facilities." This reply is the SHEER OSTRACIZATION of which I spoke of earlier!

Not only had the representative of the palliative care program not replied to my professional email directly, she had gone through a third party who had messaged me privately on her behalf. I do appreciate their honesty of acknowledging that treating CRPS is beyond their expertise. As, a reminder, treatment is not a part of palliative care. However, to deny clergy and psychological support to the patient and family is certainly NOT beyond their expertise. It is the foundation of this discipline. It was simply denied leaving an exhausted warrior, once again, utterly alone in her fight.

This is ostracizing people at their greatest time of need. To add further insult, it was recommended that I merely seek a peer support group! I do believe the fact that I have my own patient advocacy probably constitutes peer support! Much physical and emotional energy went into this communication to be met with a patronizing, insulting and outright cruel response from the medical community itself - a part of the medical community dedicated to relieving suffering and offering comfort and dignity no less. This the epitome of the ostracization and discrimination of CRPS patients (and other chronic illness warriors) I seek to eliminate for us all.

I hope and pray that one day soon I will see a resurgence of patient centered care. I am thankful for the upsurge in telehealth, this has been a wonderful step of progress. I will continue to advocate with physicians, City leaders, the AAHCM (American Academy of Home Care Medicine) and other advocacy groups for physician house call accessibility for everyone in need.

The Mayo Clinic and other huge medical entities have begun a "hospital at home" program. This will provide the same basic benefits of a hospital stay in the comfort of one's home! It is offered in very limited metro areas at this time. It is a wonderful initiative. I am following it closely.

MEDICAL CARE SHOULD BE AS ACCESSIBLE TO THE ILL AS IT IS TO THE WELL.

This is the story of how "Shannon's Hope for House Calls & Home Care" was born. I hope to have the strength to manage a website soon. I am forever reaching out to local physicians hoping to reach a provider who is willing and has the heart to care for the zebras of the world even if the hoofbeats sound like a horse.

NO ONE SHOULD BE DENIED CARE OR SUPPORT DUE TO THEIR MEDICAL DIAGNOSIS.

This has been, and continues to be, an incredibly rewarding and cathartic journey. One which I am most grateful to have taken the first step toward in December of 2019. I am here to initiate hope for all others living this struggle. May my experiences pave a new path of home-based medical care to all in need. This is my aspiration and prayer. NEVER GIVE UP. NERVER!

My story is one of survival. The literal fight to survive. Survival when the only person in this fight was myself. May we all have a future of hope from the struggles! Shannon E. Killebrew

Shannon's Hope for House Calls and Home Medical Care
Statesboro, GA. U.S.A
shannonshopehc@gmail.com
Facebook: "Shannon's Hope for House Calls and Home Medical Care"
Instagram: "shannons.hope"

"Meeting People at THEIR Level of Need."

CRPS INFORMATION RESOURCE PAGE

CRPS education, and awareness are very important to patients and their family members.

Through education, awareness, and research maybe someday we can find a cure for CRPS?

For more helpful information on CRPS, please visit The International RSD Foundation at: **www.rsdinfo.com**

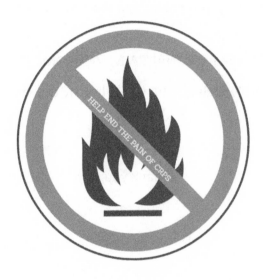

CRPS AWARNESS MONTH

November is CRPS Awareness Month!

Please tell your family and friends that November is CRPS Awareness Month. It is important for us to celebrate CRPS Awareness Month, to help spread more awareness, and provide more education about this painful disease.

Please Write A Book Review On Amazon!

We would appreciate if you could take the time to write a review about this book:

COMPLEX REGIONAL PAIN SYNDROME (CRPS):

PATIENTS' PERSPECTIVE OF LIVING IN CHRONIC PAIN
Volume V

Thank you,

Sincerely,

Doctor Al and Eric